WORKBOOK
for
PRINCIPLES AND PRACTICE OF VETERINARY TECHNOLOGY

Third Edition

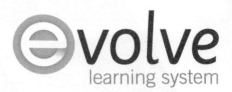

learning system

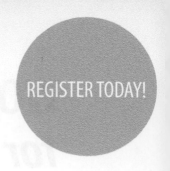

To access your Student Resources, visit:

http://evolve.elsevier.com/Sirois/principles

Register today and gain access to:

Complete downloadable image collection from the book

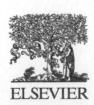

WORKBOOK
for
PRINCIPLES AND PRACTICE OF VETERINARY TECHNOLOGY

Third Edition

Margi Sirois, EdD, MS, RVT, LAT
Program Director, Veterinary Technician Program
Penn Foster College
Scottsdale, Arizona

With 125 figures

3251 Riverport Lane
St Louis, Missouri 63146

WORKBOOK FOR PRINCIPLES AND PRACTICE
OF VETERINARY TECHNOLOGY

978-0-323-07790-3

ISBN 978-0-323-07790-3

Vice President and Publisher: Linda Duncan
Publisher: Penny Rudolph
Managing Editor: Teri Merchant
Publishing Services Manager: Julie Eddy
Project Manager: Marquita Parker
Design Direction: Charlie Seibel

Contributors

Wilma P. Abbott, CVT
Adjunct Faculty
Veterinary Technology, Penn Foster College
Scottsdale, AZ
Senior Veterinary Technician/Hospital Administrator
Raccoon Valley Animal Hospital, Mullica Hill, New Jersey

Carrie Jo Anderson, CVT
Instructor, Veterinary Technology Program
Hillsborough Community College
Plant City, Florida;
Surgical Technician
Florida Veterinary Specialists, Tampa, Florida

Marg Brown, RVT, BEd AD ED
Former Professor, Veterinary Technician Program
Seneca College, King Campus
King City, Ontario;
Adjunct Faculty
Penn Foster College, Scottsdale, Arizona

Mary Tefend Campbell, CVT, VTS (ECC)
Carriage Hills Veterinary Referral Hospital
Montgomery, Alabama

Markiva Contris, LVT, BA
Professor, Veterinary Technology
Pierce College, Lakewood, Washington

Sharyn Niskala, CVT, RVT, LVT
Instructor, Veterinary Technology
Brevard Community College
Cocoa, Florida
Lead Certified Technician, Surgery
VCA Village Animal Hospital
Palm Bay, Florida

Katie Samuelson, DVM
Adjunct Faculty
Veterinary Technician Program
Penn Foster College
Scottsdale, AZ

Margi Sirois, EdD, MS, RVT, LAT
Program Director, Veterinary Technician Program
Penn Foster College
Scottsdale, Arizona

Teresa Sonsthagen, BS, LVT
Veterinary Technologist
Animal Science
North Dakota State University
Fargo, North Dakota

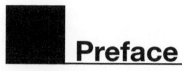

Preface

This workbook is intended to accompany the third edition of the textbook *Principles and Practice of Veterinary Technology*. Each chapter in the workbook relates to a corresponding chapter in the textbook and stresses the essential information of the chapter through the use of definitions, short essays (comprehension), photo quizzes, matching, completion, true and false, multiple choice questions, word searches, crosswords, and superclues.

Learning objectives are included at the beginning of each chapter to help you focus on the material and concepts that you are expected to learn and how this is to be applied in the veterinary clinical setting.

The following suggestions will help you use this workbook to identify strengths and weaknesses.

1. Review the contents of each chapter before you attempt to do the exercise. Do not treat the questions individually and then refer to the text for the correct answer. Deal with the chapter's subject matter as a whole, since many of the questions are interrelated. This is a learning exercise meant to help you learn the material presented in the textbook, not an examination for grades.

2. Remember that the same subject matter may be repeated in different question forms in each chapter or other chapters, since the material overlaps. The subjects of the questions are not in the same order as they appear in the textbook.

3. Read each question and study each illustration carefully before answering. You may know the answer or you may arrive at the correct answer by knowing which answers are incorrect.

4. This workbook is designed so that the pages can be easily removed, submitted if required, and placed in your notebook with the corresponding lecture notes.

The answers to all the exercises appear in the back of the book and in the Instructor Resources for *Principles and Practice of Veterinary Technology* on the Evolve website.

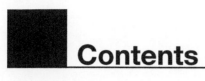

Contents

Contents

1 Overview of Veterinary Technology

LEARNING OBJECTIVES

After reviewing this chapter, the reader will be able to:
- Outline education of veterinary technicians
- Define appropriate nomenclature describing veterinary personnel
- Identify veterinary technician duties
- Differentiate between certification, registration, and licensing
- Compare career opportunities and salary ranges
- Recognize professional organizations supporting veterinary technicians
- Determine who can become a Veterinary Technician Specialist (VTS)
- Define trends in veterinary technology

TRUE OR FALSE

1. _____ The employing veterinarian has the ultimate responsibility for using a veterinary technician in an appropriate ethical manner, consistent with state and federal law.

2. _____ For a reasonable annual fee, membership in The Veterinary Support Personnel Network allows technicians to participate in online continuing education, live chats, and surveys.

3. _____ A society has bylaws, leaders, and committees designed to oversee technician specialty certification.

4. _____ Veterinary Technology is the science and art of providing professional support to veterinarians.

5. _____ For many years, consultants have cautioned veterinarians against delegating technical tasks to veterinary technicians.

6. _____ In the 2007 NAVTA national survey, 34.2% of respondents had a baccalaureate degree.

7. _____ Veterinary Technicians that maintain their certification, registration, or license after passing the VTNE are referred to as credentialed veterinary technicians.

8. _____ Approximately 1840 veterinary technicians graduated from AVMA accredited programs in 2008.

9. _____ Team efficiency improves and benchmark standards are achieved when veterinary practice management is doctor centered.

10. _____ Veterinarians delegate many income-producing procedures to veterinary technicians.

FILL IN THE BLANK

1. AVMA-accredited veterinary technology programs must design curricula that ensure each student performs all essential tasks listed in the _____.

2. Upon graduation from an AVMA-accredited veterinary technology program, candidate veterinary technicians are eligible to take the _____.

3. The _____ owns and administers the VTNE.

4. Technician _____ is typically maintained by a private or professional organization (e.g., a state veterinary technician association) and is often voluntary.

5. Duties of the _____ may include restraining, feeding, and exercising patients, cleaning the hospital and boarding premises, and other clinical support tasks.

1

6. To attain AVMA accreditation, veterinary technology education programs must meet 11 minimum requirements pertaining to facilities, faculty, _____, and _____.

7. The _____ offers economic benchmarking resources and can help veterinary technicians understand business profit or loss and budgeting.

8. In most cases, graduates of AVMA-accredited programs in veterinary technology are granted a/an _____ degree.

9. By veterinary practice law, veterinary technicians and technologists are unable to diagnose, _____, or perform surgery.

10. _____ is an online tool offering region-specific cost of living and salary information for veterinary technicians.

SHORT ANSWER

1. What types of veterinary technician credentials are usually maintained by the state government, veterinary state board, or veterinary technician association?

_____

2. How does the American Veterinary Medical Association define veterinary technicians?

_____

_____

3. What group oversees the specialty academies credentialing veterinary technician specialists?

_____

4. How can veterinary technicians advance the cause for better utilization of veterinary technicians, attain greater professional recognition, and develop more effective continuing education programs?

_____

_____

_____

5. What veterinary technicians are eligible to become veterinary technician specialists?

_____

_____

6. How are technician assistants or veterinary assistants generally trained in job duties?

_____

7. How has the general public become more aware of the role of veterinary technicians and the skilled, compassionate care they provide to family pets, companion animals, and livestock?

_____

_____

8. What does the National Association of Veterinary Technicians in America consider a cornerstone in the effective delivery of veterinary medicine?

_____

9. Name some resources found at the NAVTA website.

_____

_____

10. What benefits are seen when veterinary technology students complete an internship at a veterinary hospital?

_____

_____

LISTS

1. List seven possible members of the veterinary team:

    1. _____

    2. _____

    3. _____

    4. _____

    5. _____

    6. _____

    7. _____

2. List seven clinical pathology duties of the veterinary technician:

    1. _____

    2. _____

    3. _____

    4. _____

    5. _____

    6. _____

    7. _____

3. List five nonpractice career opportunities for veterinary technicians:

    1. _____

    2. _____

    3. _____

    4. _____

    5. _____

4. Identify six trends anticipated in veterinary technology:

1. _____

2. _____

3. _____

4. _____

5. _____

6. _____

5. List six duties of the veterinary technician when caring for hospitalized patients:

1. _____

2. _____

3. _____

4. _____

5. _____

6. _____

MATCHING

Match the group with its purpose.

_____ 1. Academy

_____ 2. CVTEA

_____ 3. Society

A. Committee of the AVMA that accredits veterinary technician programs
B. Association of professionals with common interests
C. Specialty group involved in credentialing of individuals

Match the team member with the description.

_____ 1. Veterinary Assistant

_____ 2. Veterinary Technician

_____ 3. Veterinary Technologist

_____ 4. Veterinary Technician Specialist

_____ 5. Veterinarian

A. A person who has graduated from a 2-year AVMA-accredited program
B. A person who has graduated from a 4-year CVTEA-accredited program
C. A person with the training of a clinical aide (less than that required of a veterinary technician)
D. A person who has graduated from a 4-year AVMA-accredited program receiving a Doctor of Veterinary Medicine degree
E. Credentialed technician who meets requirements established by an academy

CROSSWORD PUZZLE

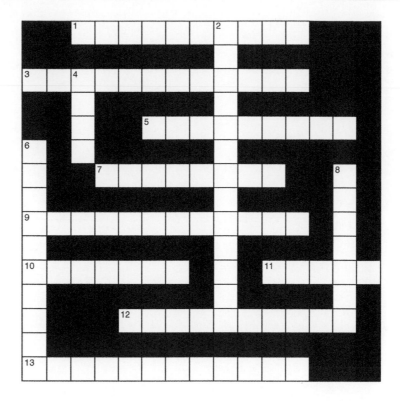

Across

1 A veterinary __ has graduated from a 2-year AVMA-accredited program. (10)

3 A person with a DVM degree. (12)

5 A veterinary __ is a person with the training of a clinical aide, which is less than that required of a veterinary technician. (9)

7 The veterinary __ act is the law governing veterinary medicine in a state. (8)

9 A __ veterinary technician is a person who has graduated from an AVMA-accredited program, passed the VTNE, and maintains certification, registration, or licensure in the state in which he/she lives. (12)

10 Establishes its own bylaws, leaders, and application, testing, and credentialing committees and tests only those candidates who meet specific requirements. (7)

11 Acronym for the group of individuals from varying backgrounds who oversee the curricula and guidelines set forth by AVMA. (5)

12 Veterinary __ is the science and art of providing professional support service to veterinarians. (10)

13 A veterinary __ has graduated from a 4-year AVMA-accredited program. (12)

Down

2 Generally kept by a private or professional organization like a state veterinary technician association. (13)

4 The veterinary __ consists of a veterinarian, veterinary technician, assistants, receptionists, and hospital managers. (4)

6 A veterinary technician __ is credentialed and has met all the requirements established by a testing agency and passed an exam according to an organization's guidelines. (10)

8 A group consisting of a general membership of people with a common interest in a veterinary technician discipline. (7)

2 Ethical, Legal, and Safety Issues in Veterinary Medicine

LEARNING OBJECTIVES

After reviewing this chapter, the reader will be able to:
- Discuss ethical issues and guidelines relevant to the veterinary profession
- Describe the veterinary technician Code of Ethics
- List and describe general categories of laws relevant to the veterinary profession
- Define laws protecting veterinary employees against physical injury, sexual harassment, and discrimination
- Explain laws relating to ensuring quality veterinary service
- Define laws regulating in the biomedical industry and Occupational Health Safety related to research
- Identify mechanisms to avoid hazards in the veterinary workplace
- Identify primary zoonotic diseases that pose a danger to veterinary personnel
- Describe procedures to minimize exposure to ionizing radiation and compressed gases
- Describe methods to prevent the spread of infectious diseases
- Discuss the content and uses of Material Safety Data Sheets
- Identify four biosafety hazard levels and precautions for each

SHORT ANSWER

1. Where are state laws for the veterinary profession outlined and recorded?

   _____

   _____

2. Why should clients not be allowed to restrain their pet during exam or treatment by the veterinarian?

   _____

   _____

3. Why might portable x-ray machines be considered particularly dangerous?

   _____

   _____

4. Identify the two sources of federal law on the care and use of animals in the biomedical industry.

   _____

   _____

5. How can the chance of slip and fall injuries in the veterinary facility be reduced?

   _____

   _____

6. When handling specimens such as fecal samples, laboratory samples, or wound exudates, what minimum safety precautions should a veterinary technician use?

   _____

   _____

7. What special precautions should a veterinary technician take when treating animals with diseases that are infectious to people or other animals?

_____

_____

8. Name one function of a code of ethics.

_____

_____

9. Name two bacterial infections transmitted to pets and humans by ticks.

_____

_____

_____

10. What guidelines are provided by OSHA's Right to Know Law?

_____

_____

_____

11. What state government group, composed of veterinary and nonveterinary professionals, is responsible for interpreting law and standards of care offered to veterinary patients?

_____

_____

12. A legal obligation of the veterinary hospital is to competently render specific services contracted with a pet owner. Beyond that, what moral responsibility does the veterinary hospital have?

_____

13. When is ordinary negligence subject to legal action?

_____

14. What forms of sex discrimination are made illegal by federal law?

_____

_____

15. What does the Comprehensive Drug Abuse Prevention and Control Act do?

_____

_____

_____

MATCHING

Match the following terms with their description or definition.

_____ 1. Human-Animal Bond

_____ 2. Drug Enforcement Agency

_____ 3. Collimator

_____ 4. Biosafety Level III Agents

_____ 5. Ringworm

_____ 6. National Institutes of Health

_____ 7. Laws

_____ 8. Fair Labor Standard Act

_____ 9. Standard Operating Procedure

_____ 10. Biosafety Level IV Agents

_____ 11. Ethics

_____ 12. Common Law

_____ 13. Biosafety Level II Agents

_____ 14. Dosimetry Badge

_____ 15. Biosafety Level I Agents

A. Maximum limits from which we can deviate from the acceptable norm

B. System of moral principles that determine behavior

C. A body of unwritten law—evolved from use, custom, and judicial decisions—that establishes precedential case law

D. Enforces federal law on the care and use of animals in the biomedical industry

E. Ordinarily do not cause disease in humans but may affect individuals with immune deficiency

F. Have potential to cause human disease if handled incorrectly; low potential for aerosol transmission

G. Can cause serious and potentially lethal disease; potential for aerosol respiratory transmission is high

H. Pose a high risk of causing life-threatening disease

I. Superficial skin infection caused by a fungus, easily transmitted from animals to humans

J. Radiation safety device found on the x-ray machine, restricts size of primary x-ray beam

K. Radiation safety device, measures personal scatter radiation exposure

L. Concept defining the special, healthy relationship between people and pets

M. Establishes minimum wage, overtime, recordkeeping, and youth employment standards

N. Primary federal law enforcement agency responsible for combating the abuse of controlled drugs

O. An official detailed description of how each important procedure should be performed at a research facility

FILL IN THE BLANK

1. Veterinary technicians should recruit help when lifting patients weighing more than _____ pounds.

2. Ethics are based on _____ principles rather than on the minimum requirements of the law.

3. _____ is empowered to address every aspect of animal use, including review of specific research that will be conducted, housing of animals, enrichment plans, pain management, and training of research personnel.

4. Never place _____ between a large animal and the side of an enclosure, stock, or chute.

5. Noise levels in canine wards can reach _____ decibels.

6. Large cylinders of compressed gas should strapped to a _____ when moved.

7. Detailed information regarding content, handling, and hazards of every chemical found in a veterinary office is located in the _____.

8. Some species of _____ larvae can migrate to virtually any organ in the body and develop into an unnoticed cystlike growth, which may be problematic in vital organs.

9. Sharps (needles, scalpel blades) must be disposed of in _____.

10. Chemical spill sites and contaminated equipment should be washed with _____, unless its use is prohibited by the instructions on the MSDS.

Chapter 2 Ethical, Legal, and Safety Issues in Veterinary Medicine

1. List three dangers associated with long-term exposure to waste anesthetic gases:

    1. _____

    2. _____

    3. _____

2. List four pieces of personal protective equipment that should be used when taking radiographs:

    1. _____

    2. _____

    3. _____

    4. _____

3. List five items that may be covered by medical waste management laws:

    1. _____

    2. _____

    3. _____

    4. _____

    5. _____

4. List six types of biomedical companies and institutions that employ veterinary technicians:

    1. _____

    2. _____

    3. _____

    4. _____

    5. _____

    6. _____

5. Formaldehyde is a known human carcinogen. List four recommendations or precautions that should be taken when handling it in the veterinary facility:

    1. _____

    2. _____

    3. _____

    4. _____

6. What are the four categories of laws that govern practice within a veterinary clinic?

    1. _____

    2. _____

    3. _____

    4. _____

7. Name the three elements a plaintiff must prove to establish that malpractice has occurred:

1. _____

2. _____

3. _____

8. Federal Equal Employment Opportunity laws prevent discrimination by employers in hiring or firing practices on the basis of what criteria?

1. _____

2. _____

3. _____

4. _____

5. _____

9. Name three laws enforced by the U.S. Fish and Wildlife Service and the Department of the Interior that may come into play when research requires the capture of animals from the wild:

1. _____

2. _____

3. _____

10. Identify four items that a biomedical industry institution should include in an Occupational Safety and Health Program:

1. _____

2. _____

3. _____

4. _____

MATCHING

Match the following.

_____ 1. Comprehensive Drug Abuse Prevention and Control Act

_____ 2. Controlled Substance Act (CSA)

_____ 3. Department of Labor

_____ 4. Drug Enforcement Agency

_____ 5. Occupational Safety and Health Act

_____ 6. Animal Welfare Act

_____ 7. Centers for Disease Control and Prevention

_____ 8. American Association for Laboratory Animal Science

A. Law most applicable to the veterinary community regarding the drugs used by veterinarians

B. Law created in 1970 by the U.S. Congress to regulate the manufacturing distribution, dispensing, and delivery of certain drugs that have the potential for abuse

C. Involved in developing and applying disease prevention and control, environment health, and health promotion and education activities designed to improve the health of the people in the United States

D. Federal law designed to provide a safe workplace for all persons working in any business affecting commerce

E. Federal agency that fosters and promotes welfare of job seekers, wage earners, and retirees, administering a variety of labor laws including those that guarantee workers' rights to safe and healthful working conditions

F. Organization dedicated to the humane care and treatment of laboratory animals and the quality research that leads to scientific gains that benefit people and animals

G. Primary federal law enforcement agency responsible for combating the abuse of controlled drugs

H. Regulates the treatment of animals in research, exhibition, transport, and by dealers

Chapter 2 **Ethical, Legal, and Safety Issues in Veterinary Medicine**

Identify the term described and then find the words in the Word Search.

1. Containing or being poisonous, especially when capable of causing death or serious debilitation

   _____

2. Any substance, radionuclide, or radiation that is an agent directly involved in the promotion of cancer or in the increase of its propagation _____

3. Capable of being transmitted from animals to human beings _____

4. Material Safety Data Sheet _____

5. Wide range of medicinal products created by biologic processes (as opposed to chemically)

   _____

6. Identifying if a health care provider fell below the level of competence expected of the professional

   _____

7. Type of negligence in which a health care provider fails to follow generally accepted professional standards, causing injury to the patient _____

8. The system of moral principles that determines appropriate behavior and actions within a specific group

   _____

9. Concerned with principles of right and wrong or conforming to standards of behavior and character based on those principles _____

10. Occupational Safety and Health Act _____

11. Drug Enforcement Agency _____

12. Controlled Substance Act _____

13. American Association for Laboratory Animal Science _____

14. Standard Operational Procedure _____

15. Personal protective equipment _____

```
N  E  G  O  N  I  C  R  A  C  X  E  P  P
J  E  H  M  S  D  Y  F  K  U  U  T  X  V
W  D  G  L  K  H  T  O  W  Z  O  H  P  D
D  S  A  L  F  S  A  G  B  T  Q  I  Y  E
F  G  C  P  I  Q  Q  V  L  A  S  C  G  A
C  A  Y  I  D  G  T  E  Q  L  L  S  F  X
C  S  I  T  G  O  E  V  Y  H  U  T  G  P
I  H  O  G  D  O  P  N  B  S  D  S  M  I
X  N  P  W  R  X  L  M  C  B  R  H  U  U
O  K  O  X  U  T  K  O  I  E  X  S  V  O
T  Q  S  A  L  A  A  F  I  S  R  L  P  S
B  R  P  S  P  U  F  W  J  B  Q  A  T  H
C  I  T  O  N  O  O  Z  Y  P  X  R  R  A
Z  A  I  H  O  J  W  P  T  W  R  O  X  U
X  E  C  I  T  C  A  R  P  L  A  M  E  M
```

Chapter 2   Ethical, Legal, and Safety Issues in Veterinary Medicine

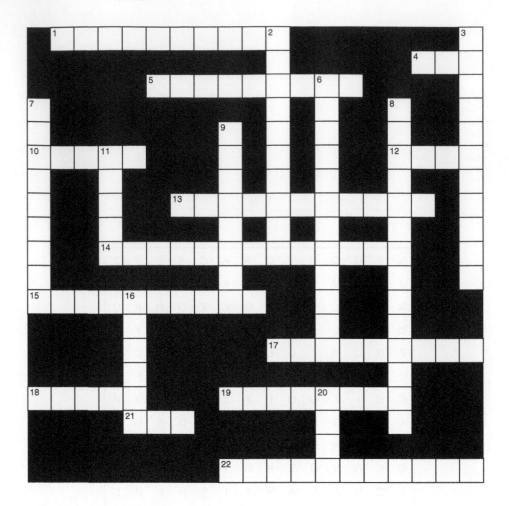

Across

1 Any agent that is directly involved in promoting cancer or increasing its propagation. (10)

4 The acronym for the primary federal law enforcement agency responsible for combating the abuse of controlled drugs. (3)

5 The wide range of medicinal products created by non-chemical processes like biotechnology and other technologies. (9)

10 The organization that is dedicated to the humane care and treatment of laboratory animals. (5)

12 The acronym for a federal law designed to provide a safe workplace for all persons working in any business effecting commerce. (4)

13 The bond that refers, for example, to the interaction between people and their pets. (2 words) (11)

14 The federal act that regulates the treatment of animals in research, exhibition, transport, and by dealers in the United States. (2 words) (13)

15 The system found on anesthetic machines that will properly discard excess anesthetic gas. (10)

17 A _____ badge is used for monitoring cumulative exposure to ionizing radiation. (9)

18 A poisonous material capable of causing death or serious debilitation. (5)

19 _____ oxide is a carcinogenic compound used to sterilize substances that would be damaged by high temperatures. (8)

21 The acronym for an official detailed description of how each important procedure should be performed at any given place of employment. (3)

22 The form of ultramicroscopic solid or liquid particles dispersed or suspended in air or gas. (11)

Down

2 When a doctor's level of competence falls below the level expected of the profession. (10)

3 A type of negligence in which a doctor fails to follow generally accepted professional standards resulting in injury to a patient. (11)

6 Education tools explaining treatments, procedures, anesthesia, risks, and the possibility of death. (2 words) (12)

7 The Board of Veterinary _____ is charged with protecting consumers and their pets and livestock. (9)

8 _____ II infectious agents have the potential to cause human disease if handled incorrectly. (2 words) (14)

9 The aqueous form of formaldehyde. (8)

11 Acronym for the group founded in 1866 that created laws against cruelty to animals. (5)

16 The system of moral principles that determines appropriate behavior and actions within a specific group. (6)

20 They set the maximum limits from which we can deviate from the acceptable norm. (4)

Chapter 2   Ethical, Legal, and Safety Issues in Veterinary Medicine

3 Practice Management

LEARNING OBJECTIVES

After reviewing this chapter, the reader will be able to:
- Identify common forms used in veterinary practice
- Describe the importance of informed consent
- Clarify admitting and discharge instructions
- Identify effective professional discharge sheets
- Describe procedures used to collect outstanding accounts
- Define and educate clients regarding pet health insurance
- Define AAHA guidelines and accreditation procedures
- Describe and comply with the Fair Labor and Standards Act
- Identify a completed medical record
- Identify and use POMR and SOAP record formats
- Identify methods used to accurately and efficiently maintain inventory
- Calculate inventory markup and cost of services
- Identify areas of and decrease loss of inventory
- Record controlled substances in appropriate log books
- Develop a disaster and recovery plan for a practice

FILL IN THE BLANK

1. An efficient, mature organization comes from managers learning to _____ and empower team members.

2. Properly operating equipment requires that team members be _____ on how it operates, which greatly extends the _____ of the equipment.

3. To prevent the purchase of excess materials _____ _____ quantities should be developed for each product.

4. Sales representatives from manufacturers have _____ developed that can explain diseases, which enhances every team member's skills.

5. The _____ _____ _____ Association provides high-quality continuing education throughout the year for hospital managers.

6. In order to put _____ at ease, a warm welcome and accessibility from team members is a must.

7. The client's experience starts with the first _____, and ends when the practice has _____ up with the visit.

8. If the client has to call the practice to receive test results, this can leave a _____ impression.

9. Receptionists should answer the phone within _____ rings.

10. Information can be misinterpreted, especially over the phone. Therefore a pet's condition must never be _____ over the phone!

11. A recommendation given to a client over the phone must be _____ in the medical record.

12. Appointment schedules should be developed to _____ production, while _____ client wait time.

13. The U.S. Department of Agriculture issues _____ _____ by the state and requires that a veterinarian do a physical exam on the animal before signing it.

14. Horses are required to have a current negative status for _____ in order to travel between states.

15. When the receptionist details the entire _____ for the client, it shows the total value of the visit.

16. Accounts receivable totals should never exceed _____ % of the total gross revenue amount.

17. In order for district attorneys to prosecute bad check writers, a _____ number must be written on the check.

18. A collection agency's report can remain on a client's credit report for _____ years; therefore they are willing to pay the debt.

19. Patients discharged from the hospital must be released with _____ instructions.

20. Discharging instructions should be given and payment should be made (**before/after**) the pet is brought to the client. (circle one)

21. The increased use of pet _____ is expected to decrease the number of euthanasias performed each year because of cost of medical services.

22. Indemnity insurance offers _____ for treatment of injured and sick pets.

23. A _____ is defined as the amount an owner pays monthly or annually to maintain an insurance policy for their pet.

24. A _____ is the amount an owner must pay before the insurance company will offer compensation.

25. A co-pay is the _____ that the owner is responsible for after the deductible has been met.

26. Insurance may be denied because of a _____ condition which is an abnormality transmitted by genes from parent to offspring.

27. The cost of hiring and training a new employee can equal at least _____ year's salary.

28. **True or False** (circle one) During an interview the candidate can be asked if she is planning to have children.

29. A written job description and the hospital _____ are important parts of training a new employee.

30. Rewards and recognition of employees should be made _____, and reprimands and

    corrections should be done _____.

31. All employees are to be paid an hourly wage except if the employee holds a _____ degree or is

    an _____ assistant.

32. Any employee working more than _____ hours within 1 work week must be paid overtime at 1½ times the regular rate of pay.

33. Employee records should be kept for at least _____ years after the employee has left the practice.

34. A medical record is a legal document that must be maintained for _____ years if the client has not returned to the practice.

35. If computerized records are used, _____ accuracy is necessary for all data entry; incorrectly entered computer records may never be retrieved.

36. The most common error made is not documenting the communication with the owner regarding the _____ of the patient.

37. A goal for the inventory manager is to not exceed the average shelf life of an item, which is _____ months.

38. The number of times inventory turns over in a practice in a specified time is referred to as _____/ _____.

39. When a current client/patient/veterinarian relationship exists a _____ product can be sold.

40. Next to payroll, _____ is the largest expense to the practice.

41. Any loss of a controlled substance greater than _____% per year must be immediately reported to the police department, State Veterinary and/or Pharmacy Board, and the DEA.

42. When ordering a controlled substance in either class I or II, DEA form _____ must be filled out and mailed to the distributor.

43. Computers only function optimally for _____ to _____ years and then need to be replaced.

44. The practice manager is responsible for the _____ of the facility and equipment.

45. Veterinary medical personnel can receive training in disaster aid from courses by _____.

SHORT ANSWER

1. Explain why an orthopedic appointment is given more time than a yearly vaccination appointment.

_____

_____

_____

_____

2. What types of appointments can veterinary technicians handle without the veterinarian?

_____

_____

_____

_____

3. What information should be gathered and entered into the schedule—either on paper or on a computer?

_____

_____

_____

_____

4. How do reminder calls help the practice and the clients?

_____

_____

_____

_____

Chapter 3 Practice Management

5. How can dropping a pet off at the clinic be of great service to the client?

_____

_____

_____

6. How can you greet a client if you are on the phone or already helping a client?

_____

_____

_____

7. Explain why most new patient/client forms have to include a phone and driver's license number?

_____

_____

_____

_____

8. Explain what a blanket consent form is and why it is not the best form to utilize.

_____

_____

_____

_____

9. List the information that must be included on a rabies certificate.

Owner Information	Patient Information	Veterinary Information
_____	_____	_____
_____	_____	_____
	_____	_____
		_____
		_____

10. Explain how credit card machines and check verification systems work.

_____

_____

_____

_____

11. Describe what limitations the Fair Debt Collections Act place on a business that makes collection calls.

_____

_____

_____

_____

12. List some of the things the veterinary technician can educate clients about during the office visit.

_____

_____

_____

_____

13. If admitting a patient the client needs to sign some forms. What would these most likely be?

_____

_____

_____

_____

14. Why would a practice want to become AAHA accredited?

_____

_____

_____

_____

15. Why is it so important to offer vacation time to your employees?

_____

_____

_____

_____

16. What records should be kept on each employee?

_____

_____

_____

_____

17. Explain why medical records are legal documents and how they should be written to maintain the document.

_____

_____

_____

_____

18. How can you fix errors on both paper and a paperless medical record?

_____

_____

_____

_____

19. What do the acronyms POMR and SOAP stand for in regards to medical records?

_____

_____

_____

_____

20. What commonly overlooked errors and incomplete medical records can be caught by diligent team members?

_____

_____

_____

_____

21. What are SOPs and why are they so useful in the veterinary practice?

_____

_____

_____

_____

22. Describe the qualities an inventory manager should have.

_____

_____

_____

_____

23. What are the costs associated with ordering a product for the clinic?

_____

_____

_____

_____

24. Explain how to determine "turns/year" and "shelf life" numbers for inventory.

_____

_____

_____

_____

25. Give three examples of products that can only be sold by a veterinarian when a client/patient relationship exists.

_____

_____

_____

26. Describe how everyone on the team can help recover costs by using "travel sheets."

_____

_____

_____

_____

27. Rewrite this label so it is more concise: "Give 1 capsule every 8 hours."

_____

_____

28. Explain the differences between "shopped services" and "in-hospital fees."

_____

_____

_____

_____

29. How can you tell if a medication is a controlled substance?

_____

_____

30. How can computers benefit a veterinary practice?

_____

_____

_____

_____

31. How do team members learn to use management software?

_____

_____

32. Give an example of direct marketing.

_____

_____

33. Give an example of internal marketing.

_____

_____

34. What are some examples of "value-added service?"

_____

_____

35. What information must be readily available to handle a natural disaster emergency?

_____

_____

_____

_____

WORD SEARCH

Identify the term described and then find the words in the Word Search.

1. Agenda: a temporally organized plan for matters to be attended to _____

2. Arrangement for a meeting or examination _____

3. Someone who controls resources and expenditures _____

4. Animal owner; someone who pays for goods and services _____

5. Having to do with bones _____

6. In a veterinary practice, may consist of a veterinarian, technician, assistant, receptionist, and hospital managers

   _____

7. A machine that manipulates data according to a set of instructions _____

8. In veterinary practice, an animal _____

9. A drug that has been deemed by the DEA as potentially abusive _____

10. Activity leading to skilled behavior _____

11. An order from a licensed veterinarian directing a pharmacist to prepare a drug for use in a client's animal

    _____

12. Catastrophe _____

13. Deliberate plans of action to guide decisions and achieve rational outcomes _____

14. Knowledge acquired by learning and instruction _____

15. Anything providing permanent evidence of or information about past events _____

16. A worker who is hired to perform a job _____

17. A document that contains a summary or listing of relevant job experience and education _____

18. Goods used primarily in the operation of a business _____

19. A person employed to represent a business and to sell its merchandise _____

20. A detailed list of all the items in stock _____

21. Any book or register, including an electronic format, used for the purposes of recording information

    _____

```
G  M  H  R  O  G  A  S  K  P  L  L  B  T  T  E  R  J  M  Q  C  J  O  B  T
R  U  Z  J  W  H  R  A  A  A  B  W  Q  A  N  E  A  R  V  O  I  S  V  M  B
I  L  O  B  U  W  F  L  T  T  B  I  O  Y  C  M  L  V  N  Y  D  L  C  Z  C
Y  F  P  P  J  I  E  F  I  N  P  N  O  N  G  R  Z  P  S  E  E  O  W  Q
Y  A  P  L  Q  N  J  S  P  E  C  E  R  V  T  O  R  A  I  V  P  C  M  T  Z
U  S  D  T  W  P  E  R  P  N  T  D  M  W  E  O  Y  N  Z  G  O  N  P  B  P
J  E  Q  U  I  P  M  E  N  T  S  W  X  T  L  N  O  I  N  X  H  A  U  U  S
Q  L  G  K  P  X  E  P  T  I  M  M  D  E  N  I  T  I  Y  A  T  T  T  D  D
R  R  J  Z  V  C  J  R  E  M  A  Y  C  B  T  I  N  O  O  P  R  S  E  E  M
G  G  S  P  A  R  G  E  P  F  A  S  M  A  X  I  O  W  R  E  O  B  R  E  H
K  X  J  Q  Y  V  Z  S  V  F  U  N  C  O  A  P  E  P  X  Y  P  U  S  T  T
S  G  G  C  D  V  C  E  F  R  J  U  A  R  S  A  L  X  P  A  S  S  H  W  O
T  N  E  I  L  C  Y  N  S  F  D  K  T  G  H  V  U  U  G  A  B  D  N  F  H
D  D  X  T  J  F  U  T  C  E  U  S  X  T  E  U  D  Z  O  V  P  E  Q  M  K
J  N  G  Z  B  F  P  A  A  I  E  P  Y  P  P  R  E  B  S  G  C  L  A  Q  B
I  N  Q  E  A  N  N  T  N  U  L  Q  S  J  E  V  H  Y  G  G  P  L  F  I  S
S  Z  L  H  C  R  J  I  P  G  S  O  L  E  S  N  C  X  D  G  Z  O  W  Y  J
O  G  N  E  Y  J  N  V  R  O  M  T  U  F  I  O  S  I  G  Y  T  R  D  L  L
E  E  Y  O  L  P  M  E  N  O  I  T  P  I  R  C  S  E  R  P  E  T  F  G  M
J  M  A  A  E  U  N  K  Q  U  L  B  O  P  S  A  I  P  F  A  I  N  T  P  A
H  L  U  P  U  X  K  K  K  E  Q  C  N  L  S  H  F  L  O  G  B  O  O  K  E
K  K  M  S  J  W  K  R  I  P  T  I  U  T  E  J  S  Z  O  V  Z  C  A  Z  T
D  I  W  L  E  R  Z  L  N  M  T  T  E  T  K  K  T  H  N  P  C  X  M  M  C
K  L  H  T  N  R  H  H  J  C  H  R  F  Y  L  J  W  N  J  Y  Q  G  M  V  L
M  X  Q  E  C  X  F  W  G  F  J  M  E  C  A  B  K  C  H  O  B  V  E  R  O
```

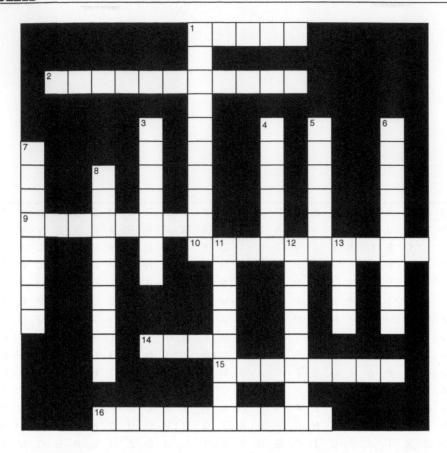

Across

1 The specified dollar amount of a covered service that is the policyholder's responsibility. (5)

2 __ accounts are the monies owed to a veterinary practice by clients. (11)

9 The time worked after having worked 40 hours in 1 week. (8)

10 The fee that is added to prescriptions to cover the cost of the pill vial, label, and team member's time. (10)

14 The acronym for the most commonly used medical record format followed by veterinary health care teams. (4)

15 The __ order quantity is an equation used to determine the correct amount of inventory to order. (8)

16 The dollar amount an individual must pay for services prior to the insurance company's payment. (10)

Down

1 A __ substance is a drug that has been deemed susceptible to abuse by the DEA. (10)

3 The amount paid for a policyholder to maintain an insurance policy. (7)

4 Pricing a product based on a percentage of cost, such as per tablet, per milliliter, or per bottle. (6)

5 The difference between the selling price and the cost per unit. (6)

6 __ insurance is a type of insurance where the client is reimbursed for services after they have been provided. (9)

7 When a decision is made after all the facts have been presented, it is based on __ consent. (8)

8 Unexplained inventory losses. (9)

11 __ marketing is the type of marketing utilized by practices by providing clean facilities, genuine service, and excellent customer care. (8)

12 __ marketing is a marketing technique that targets potential clients. (8)

13 The acronym that indentifies the most common data entry formats used in veterinary medicine. (4)

Effective Communication in Veterinary Practice

LEARNING OBJECTIVES

After reviewing this chapter, the reader will be able to:
- Discuss methods to implement effective communication skills in the veterinary clinic
- Identify barriers that prevent successful communication exchanges
- Implement effective listening skills to enhance clinical expertise
- Implement assertive communication techniques to replace ineffective speech habits and solve conflict situations more successfully
- Review techniques to reduce conflict and manage difficult situations with team members
- Describe the stages of grief
- Explain the importance of the human-animal bond to client and coworker interaction
- Describe appropriate ways to counsel clients on loss of a companion animal

MATCHING

Match each stage of grief with its description.

_____ 1. Denial

_____ 2. Bargaining

_____ 3. Anger

_____ 4. Guilt

_____ 5. Sorrow

_____ 6. Resolution

A. Blame directed at the veterinarian, staff members, or client themselves
B. Sadness, and perhaps release of days or weeks of pent-up emotions
C. A coping mechanism that cushions the mind against the shock it has received
D. Realization that the pet is gone, nothing will change that, and client will survive this loss
E. Unproductive, unreasonable feeling of responsibility that may inhibit progress toward resolution of the loss
F. A way of keeping hope alive and buying time to fully accept the outcome of the situation

Match the following terms with their definition.

_____ 1. Compounded loss

_____ 2. Action steps

_____ 3. Empathetic listening

_____ 4. Body language

_____ 5. Assertive communication

A. Communicating without judgment, demonstrating caring and understanding
B. Communication with focus on speaking in a positive and proactive manner
C. Use of eyes, gestures, and body in conveying a message
D. A list version of exactly what must occur to resolve a conflict
E. Situation where a client facing the loss of a pet is reminded of losses from the past

TRUE OR FALSE

1. _____ As a veterinary technician, your success in practice will be based solely on technical expertise.

2. _____ The goal of communication is to exchange thoughts and ideas in a flowing, two-way manner.

3. _____ How co-workers ignore conflict situations can ultimately define their success in the veterinary practice.

4. _____ Veterinary technicians should be familiar with the stages of grief in order to recognize how clients are progressing through the stages and assist them when appropriate.

5. _____ Good listening skills will facilitate communication among co-workers.

6. _____ The grieving process is a steady, linear ascent from depression to joy.

ORDER

1. Place the following steps, which integrate assertiveness into your communication style, in chronological order (1-8):

   _____ Determine how to establish assertive communication.

   _____ Adapt this process to your style; remember it in the future.

   _____ Recognize negative tendencies and the barricade they represent.

   _____ Determine what needs to be said, set your goal, take initiative to initiate the interaction.

   _____ Know what you want.

   _____ Review what happened and what you can learn from this interaction.

   _____ Challenge negative tendencies and replace them with positive thoughts.

   _____ Pat yourself on the back.

FILL IN THE BLANK

1. Mastering _____ improves both client and co-worker interactions.

2. The active listener is often the _____ of the conversation.

3. _____ impact a discussion in a negative manner and increase the chance that collaboration will not occur.

4. Active listening requires _____ and _____.

5. _____ is a subcategory of nonverbal communication.

6. The first step in reducing the impact of communication barriers is to _____ them.

7. A positive resolution environment is created by the _____, the time, and the demonstration of commitment by all parties involved.

8. The veterinary team's responsibility is to help the animal, _____, and serve the client.

9. When facing the loss of a pet, clients often look to the veterinary technician for _____, assurance, _____, and validation.

10. An open posture with uncrossed arms and legs demonstrates to clients that you are _____.

LISTS

1. List the four primary methods of communication:

   1. _____

   2. _____

   3. _____

   4. _____

2. List the three categories of barriers to communication:

   1. _____

   2. _____

   3. _____

3. List five items or techniques clients may use to memorialize a deceased pet and move through the bereavement process:

1. _____

2. _____

3. _____

4. _____

5. _____

4. List the five steps in a conflict resolution plan:

1. _____

2. _____

3. _____

4. _____

5. _____

CROSSWORD PUZZLE

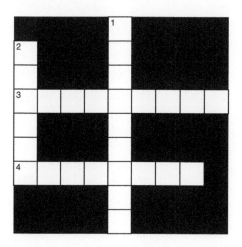

Across

3 Communication by means other than words. (9)
4 Somebody who takes delivery of something. (8)

Down

1 Communication where the person acts confidently when stating a position or claim. (9)
2 Somebody who transmits something. (6)

Chapter 4 Effective Communication in Veterinary Practice

4. List the five steps in a conflict resolution plan.

CROSSWORD PUZZLE

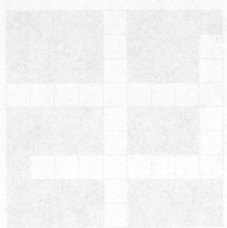

Across

3. Communication by means other than words. (9)
4. Somebody who takes delivery of something. (8)

Down

1. Communication where the people act confidently when sharing a position or claim. (9)
2. Somebody who transmits something. (6)

Veterinary Medical Terminology

LEARNING OBJECTIVES

After reviewing this chapter, the reader will be able to:
- Construct medical terms from word parts
- Describe how to construct medical terms
- Define the meanings of common prefixes and suffixes used in medical terms
- List combining forms used to refer to various body parts
- Discuss terms for direction, position, and movement
- Define terms used for common surgical procedures, diseases, instruments, procedures, and dentistry
- Name the types of cells and tissues that make up the animal body
- Name the types of bones and muscles that make up the animal body
- List and describe the components of the integument

GIVE THE MEANING

Define the following word parts.

1. ex- _____
2. hyper- _____
3. post- _____
4. dis- _____
5. per- _____
6. inter- _____
7. endo- _____
8. peri- _____
9. circum- _____
10. tachy- _____
11. –rrhea _____
12. –pathy _____
13. –pexy _____
14. –plasia _____
15. –oma _____
16. –para _____
17. –philia _____
18. –physis _____
19. –tome _____
20. colp/o _____

MATCHING

Match the meaning with the prefix/suffix.

_____ 1. -megaly

_____ 2. Ante-

_____ 3. Intra-

_____ 4. Para-

_____ 5. -crine

_____ 6. Anti-

_____ 7. -ize

_____ 8. -itis

_____ 9. Inter-

_____ 10. -osis

_____ 11. Peri-

_____ 12. Sym-

A. Against
B. Inflammation
C. Between
D. State or condition
E. Beside, apart from
F. Before
G. Within
H. Secrete
I. Around, surrounding
J. Use, subject to
K. Enlarged
L. With

FILL IN THE BLANK

Fill in the blank with the with the correct combining form.

1. Abdomen _____

2. Ankle _____

3. Chest _____

4. Diaphragm _____

5. Duct _____

6. Ear _____

7. Eye _____

8. Eyelid _____

9. Face _____

10. Fat _____

11. Foot _____

12. Gland _____

13. Hair _____

14. Lip _____

15. Mouth _____

16. Muscle _____

17. Nose _____

18. Spinal column _____

19. Spleen _____

20. Thymus gland _____

21. Toe _____

22. Tongue _____

23. Tooth _____

24. Uterus _____

25. Vein _____

Fill in the blank with the correct combining form.

1. Before birth _____

2. Without sensation or feeling _____

3. Inside the vein _____

4. Difficult breathing _____

5. Increased heart rate _____

6. Pertaining to "disease producing" _____

7. Pertaining to "throughout the entire animal kingdom" _____

8. Against coughing (cough medicine) _____

9. Lack of cells _____

10. Abnormal growth _____

11. White blood cell _____

12. Inability to move the lower body (in bipeds) or hind limbs (in quadrupeds) _____

13. Tumor of the thymus gland _____

14. Study of the endocrine system _____

15. Production of new glucose _____

16. The correct spelling for asites _____

17. The correct spelling for vulvulus _____

18. Further terms for "process" _____

19. Abnormally small eye _____

20. Pertaining to "under the shoulder blade" _____

Fill in the blank with the meaning of the word part.

1. vaso- _____

2. pseudo- _____

3. thrombo- _____

4. intra- _____

5. -ema _____

6. -stomy _____

7. -ia _____

Chapter **5** **Veterinary Medical Terminology**

8. -megaly _____

9. -penia _____

10. -phobia _____

11. -philia _____

12. -praxia _____

13. -osis _____

14. -um _____

15. olig/o _____

16. pyel/o _____

17. ureter/o _____

18. -scopy _____

19. crypt/o _____

20. dolich/o _____

Fill in the blank with the meaning of the bold underlined word part.

1. para**plegia** _____

2. hemato**crit** _____

3. **meta**stasis _____

4. macro**phage** _____

5. pro**phylaxis** _____

6. **ef**ferent _____

7. special**ize** _____

8. **vaso**genic _____

9. **cheilo**plasty _____

10. hemat**emesis** _____

Fill in the blank with the meaning of the word part.

1. macrocytosis   macro-   _____

   cyt/o   _____

   -osis   _____

2. epicarditis   epi-   _____

   cardi/o   _____

   -itis   _____

3. cardiology   cardi/o   _____

   -ology   _____

4. polydactyly   poly-   _____

                      dactyly   _____

5. congenital   con   _____

                      genit/o   _____

6. lipochondroma   lipo   _____

                      chondr/o _____

                      -oma   _____

7. antipyretic   anti-   _____

                      pyret/o   _____

                      -ic   _____

8. septicemia   septic/o   _____

                      -emia   _____

9. panzootic   pan-   _____

                      zoo   _____

10. hematuria   hemat/o   _____

                      -ur/o   _____

11. onychectomy onych/o   _____

                      -ectomy   _____

12. cardiomegaly cardi/o   _____

                      -megaly   _____

13. laparotomy   lapar/o   _____

                      -otomy   _____

14. vasculitis   vas/o   _____

                      -itis   _____

15. thoracocentesis thoraco/   _____

                      centesis   _____

1. The term for "toward the midline" is:
   a. medial
   b. lateral
   c. proximal
   d. distal

2. The paw is _____ to the shoulder.
   a. cranial
   b. caudal
   c. distal
   d. proximal

3. Another term for growth plate is:
   a. physis
   b. shaft
   c. diaphysis
   d. trophic

4. The term that describes part of the small intestine is the
   a. ileum
   b. ilium

5. Gastroplasty contains the suffix that means:
   a. excision
   b. forming an opening
   c. surgical repair
   d. incision

6. An incision into the duodenum is a:
   a. duodenectomy
   b. duodenoscopy
   c. duodenostomy
   d. duodenotomy

7. Which terms pertain to the tongue?
   a. lingual and gingival
   b. lingual and glossal
   c. lingual only
   d. gingival and glossal

8. Enteritis means inflammation of the:
   a. internal organs
   b. peritoneum
   c. small intestine
   d. esophagus

9. Mouth lacerations or cuts would most likely cause:
   a. hematemesis
   b. proteinuria
   c. polydipsia
   d. dysphagia

10. Cystotomy is:
    a. resection of the urinary bladder
    b. incision of the urinary bladder
    c. inflammation of the urinary bladder
    d. herniation of the urinary bladder

11. Polyuria:
    a. is an abbreviated way of saying renal failure
    b. is the opposite of anuria
    c. means having more than one kidney
    d. means having multiple pouches developing from the urinary bladder

12. Nephromegaly is:
    a. inflammation of the kidney
    b. suturing of the kidney
    c. constriction of the kidney
    d. enlargement of the kidney

13. Formation of a new opening into the urinary bladder is:
    a. cystostomy
    b. cystoplegia
    c. peritoneal cystogram
    d. cystotomy

14. Diaphysis is the:
    a. shaft of the long bone
    b. segment of that involves bone growth
    c. wider part of the long bone shaft
    d. wide end of the bone covered with articular cartilage

15. The term angiorrhaphy means:
    a. fixation of the vessels
    b. suturing of the vessels
    c. replacement of the vessels
    d. destruction of the vessels

16. A nasal discharge is referred to as:
    a. rhinitis
    b. rhinorrhea
    c. rhinorrhagia
    d. epistaxis

17. The surgical incision into the chest wall is known as:
    a. thoracentesis
    b. thoracostomy
    c. thoracotomy
    d. thoracectomy

18. An abnormal accumulation of blood in the pleural cavity is:
    a. hemothorax
    b. hemopleuritis
    c. hemoptysis
    d. hemopneumonia

19. The plural of fistula is:
    a. fistuli
    b. fistulae
    c. fistule
    d. fistulus

20. A benign growth of fat cells is a/an:
    a. lipoma
    b. liposarcoma
    c. adipocarcinoma
    d. adiposarcoma

21. The term for "between the toes" is:
    a. interphalangeal
    b. interdigital
    c. intraphalangeal
    d. intradigital

22. Dead tissue is said to be:
    a. necrotic
    b. plantigrade
    c. polled
    d. exfoliative

23. A malignant black tumor of skin is a/an:
    a. onychoma
    b. xanthoma
    c. adenoma
    d. melanoma

24. Deficient gland secretion is called:
    a. hypercrinism
    b. hypocrinism
    c. endocrinopathy
    d. endocrinopenia

25. Disease of the adrenal glands is termed:
    a. adrenal pathogen
    b. adrenopathy
    c. adenopathy
    d. adenosis

26. Enlargement of the thyroid gland is termed:
    a. thiromegaly
    b. thryromegaly
    c. thryomegaly
    d. thyromegaly

27. The plural of stimulus is:
    a. stimulum
    b. stimulae
    c. stimula
    d. stimuli

28. Which layer of tissue is the endometrium?
    a. middle
    b. inner
    c. outer
    d. between the outer and the peritoneum

29. The term ectopic means:
    a. in the usual location
    b. outside the usual place
    c. outside the uterus
    d. outside the reproductive system

30. Encephalomyelopathy is:
    a. hardening of brain tissue
    b. morbid softening of the brain
    c. any disease involving the brain and spinal cord
    d. any disease involving the bone marrow and skull

31. Inflammation of the outer ear is called:
    a. otitis externa
    b. otitis media
    c. otitis interna
    d. panotitis

32. An instrument used to examine the ear is a/an:
    a. oroscope
    b. ear speculum
    c. otoscope
    d. tympanospeculum

33. Incision into the cornea is called:

    a. lacromotomy

    b. keratoplasty

    c. goniotomy

    d. keratotomy

34. The correct spelling of the word meaning "bluish tinge to the skin and mucous membranes" is:

    a. cianosis

    b. cyianosis

    c. cyanosis

    d. cyanoses

35. The plural of cranium is:

    a. craniae

    b. crania

    c. cranius

    d. craniora

36. The prefix for "down under, lower, against" is:

    a. cata-

    b. andro-

    c. ana-

    d. cart-

37. Which of the following suggests "greater, excessive, beyond"

    a. hyper- or infra-

    b. super- or sub-

    c. hypo- or infra-

    d. ultra- or hypo-

38. Which of the following terms means "instrument for cutting the stomach"?

    a. gastrotomy

    b. gastrotome

    c. gastroscopy

    d. gastroscope

39. Which of the following terms means "black tumor"?

    a. xanthoma

    b. cyanoma

    c. melanoma

    d. leukoma

40. The term subcutaneous means:

    a. beneath the skin

    b. pertaining to beneath the skin

    c. abnormal condition of the skin

    d. a condition of fat

41. Which of the following terms means "partial paralysis of the stomach"?
    a. gastrodynia
    b. gastroplegia
    c. gastroparesis
    d. gastrorrhexis

42. Which of the following terms means "surgical fixation of the ureter"?
    a. ureteroplasty
    b. ureteropexy
    c. urorrhaphy
    d. ureteromegaly

43. The term nephrotomy means:
    a. surgical removal of the kidneys
    b. a mouthlike opening into the kidneys
    c. cutting into the kidneys
    d. visual examination of the kidneys

44. Dysuria means:
    a. deficient urine production
    b. painful or difficult urination
    c. blood in the urine
    d. pertaining to urination

45. Polydipsia means:
    a. decreased drinking
    b. difficult drinking
    c. no drinking
    d. much drinking

46. Based on an analysis of a urine specimen, a cat was diagnosed with a urinary tract infection. The laboratory analysis MOST likely noted:
    a. anuria
    b. oliguria
    c. pyuria
    d. nocturia

47. Osteoarthropathy means:
    a. disease of the bone and joint
    b. abnormal condition of the bone and cartilage
    c. swelling of the bone and joint
    d. destruction of the bone and cartilage

48. Parasternal means:
    a. pain in the sternum
    b. movement of the sternum
    c. around the ribs
    d. pertaining to near the sternum

49. Cystocentesis means:
    a. movement of the thorax
    b. sensation of the bladder
    c. abnormal condition of the abdomen
    d. surgical puncture of the bladder

50. The correct spelling of the word meaning "contraction of the ventricle" is:
    a. sistolle
    b. sistole
    c. systole
    d. cystole

51. Which one of the following terms is in the plural form?
    a. testis
    b. testes
    c. granuloma
    d. appendix

52. Anuric means:
    a. pertaining to absence of urine
    b. much production of urine
    c. deficiency of urine
    d. a condition of the urine

53. An abnormally rapid respiratory rate is:
    a. apnea
    b. bradypnea
    c. dyspnea
    d. tachypnea

54. Polyuria means:
    a. decreased urine production
    b. blood in the urine
    c. pain in the urethra
    d. much urine

55. Toxicology means:
    a. specialist in the study of poisons
    b. destruction of poisons
    c. study of poisons
    d. instrument for measuring poisons

56. Which of the following terms means "paralysis of the eye"?
    a. oculoplegia
    b. ophthalmoparesis
    c. otopexy
    d. blepharoptosis

57. Pyelonephritis means:
   a. specialist in the study of kidney disorders
   b. a condition of the kidneys
   c. inflammation of the renal pelvis
   d. pain in the kidneys

58. Peritoneal means:
   a. pertaining to the peritoneum
   b. a condition of the peritoneum
   c. inflammation of the peritoneum
   d. a disease of the peritoneum

59. Which of the following terms means "disease of the hair"?
   a. trichopathy
   b. pilosis
   c. trichoplasty
   d. piloslcerosis

60. The combining form kerat/o means:
   a. cornea
   b. tube
   c. sclera
   d. eye

61. Myositis means:
   a. inflammation of the muscles
   b. inflammation of the spinal cord
   c. a condition of the muscles
   d. a condition of the spinal cord
   e. pertaining to the spinal cord

62. Regarding epithelial tissue:
   a. columnar is irregular with irregular nuclei
   b. stratified cuboidal is common in the body
   c. transitional is thick and unbending
   d. squamous tissue is flat and platelike

63. With cell structure:
   a. Melanocytes produce a light pigment called melanin
   b. The sebaceous glands are the sweat glands
   c. Cattle and horses have a few, clustered sudoriferous glands in the footpad and nose
   d. Sudoriferous glands are the sweat glands

64. The arrectores pilorum muscles that attach to the hair follicles:
   a. relax as hairs are pulled more upright
   b. cool the animal
   c. is the singular while arrector pili is plural
   d. are part of the sympathetic nervous system

65. Which of the following is true regarding cartilage?
    a. consists of chondrocytes, fibers embedded in matrix and blood vessels
    b. hyaline cartilage is smooth and glossy, and makes up intervertebral discs
    c. fibrous cartilage are densely arranged collagen fibers found in trachea rings
    d. elastic cartilage is more flexibile, forming the pinna and part of the larynx

CASE STUDIES

Give the proper medical term for the boldfaced descriptions in this case study.

1. A 3-yr-old F/S DSH presented to the clinic with **blood in the urine (a)** _____ and **difficulty urinating**

   (b) _____. Urine was collected by **inserting a needle into the urinary bladder and withdrawing urine**

   (c) _____, and a **test on the urine involving breakdown of the urine components**

   (d) _____ was performed. The cat was admitted to the clinic and an ultrasound was

   performed to rule out **urinary bladder stones (e)** _____. None was evident, but tests showed an

   infection of the bladder (f) _____. The cat was placed on drugs that were effective **against life**

   (g) _____. Recheck in 10 days.

State the meaning (breaking up the word, if possible) for the boldfaced medical terms in the following case studies.

2. A 5 yr old *M/N* Doberman was presented to the clinic. After **auscultating** _____ the heart with a

   stethoscope _____, the veterinarian detected a cardiac **arrhythmia** _____, **hypoxia** _____

   with **hypercapnia** _____, and **tachycardia** _____. Radiographs revealed **cardiomegaly**

   _____, which helped to support the veterinarian's diagnosis of **cardiomyopathy** _____.

3. The veterinarian was examining a small herd of Hereford cattle that had arrived 10 days ago, after being

   transported from a large cow/calf operation. Some of the cattle have various aspects of **rhinitis** _____,

   tachypnea _____, **hyperpnea** _____, **hypopnea** _____, **dyspnea** _____, and

   cyanosis _____. The **conjunctivae** _____ were not reddened or **edema-**

   tous _____. Because of the history and respiratory signs, the veterinarian suspected bovine **pneumonic**

   _____ **pasteurellosis** _____, or shipping fever, a severe respiratory disease seen in younger ani-

   mals after shipment or stress. The affected cattle were isolated and treated with **antibiotics** _____ and a

   mucolytic _____. Management practices such as immunization and stress reduction were discussed with

   the owner so that **eupnea** _____ would soon prevail.

MATCHING

Match the bones with the descriptions in the following.

_____ 1. Long bones

_____ 2. Flat bones

_____ 3. Small bones

_____ 4. Irregular bones

_____ 5. Sesamoid bones

_____ 6. Pneumatic bones

A. Cuboidal or approximately equal in all dimensions
B. Tiny bones found along the course of the tendons
C. Contain air spaces to make the skeleton lighter
D. Expanded in two directions to provide maximum area for muscle attachment
E. Contain epiphysis and diaphysis
F. An example are vertebrae

Match the bones with the descriptions in the following.

_____ 1. Articular

_____ 2. Bone head

_____ 3. Condyle

_____ 4. Facet

_____ 5. Foramen

_____ 6. Fossa

_____ 7. Neck of bone

_____ 8. Process

A. A spherical articular projection usually found on the proximal ends of some limb bones
B. A depression in a bone usually occupied by a muscle or tendon
C. A lump or bump on the surface of a bone
D. A large, convex articular surface usually found on the distal ends of the long bones
E. Narrowed area connecting a bone head with the rest of the bone
F. A flat and smooth articular area, such as the surface of a tarsal or carpal bone
G. A hole in a bone through which blood vessels and nerves usually pass
H. Usually very smooth and often covered with a layer of hyaline cartilage

Match the vertebral formula with the correct species.

Circle the correct species for each of the following:

1. Canine, Bovine, Equine, Swine: C 7, T 13, L 7, S 3, Cy 20–23

2. Canine, Bovine, Equine, Swine: C 7, T 13, L 6, S 5, Cy 18–20

3. Canine, Bovine, Equine, Swine: C 7, T 18, L 6, S 5, Cy 15–20

TRUE OR FALSE

1. _____ Most species have one more pair of ribs than the vertebral vertebrae.

2. _____ The costal cartilages of ribs at the cranial end of the thorax are connected directly to the sternum at their ventral end.

3. _____ The manubrium sterni is the caudalmost sternebra, and the xiphoid process forms the cranial portion.

4. _____ The glenoid cavity forms the shoulder joint with the femur.

5. _____ Parts of the humerus include the head, the greater tubercle, and the condyles.

6. _____ The main weight-bearing bone of the antebrachium is the radius.

7. _____ In bovine and equine species, the radius and ulna are fused together.

8. _____ Normal synovial fluid is opaque, sticky, slippery, and viscous.

9. _____ The gastrointestinal tract is the largest body organ.

10. _____ Skeletal muscle is involuntary striated muscle.

11. _____ Myocytes are shaped like long cylinders or fibers with multiple nuclei and smaller myofibrils.

12. _____ Nerve fibers and skeletal muscle fibers connect at the musculoneural junction.

13. _____ The origin is the movable portion where skeletal muscle attaches to bone, while the insertion is the more stable attachment.

14. _____ Striated, involuntary muscles describe muscle found in hollow abdominal organs.

15. _____ Cardiac muscle cells each have an innate contractile rhythm that does not require an external nerve supply.

16. _____ Sympathetic stimulation increases the rate and force of cardiac muscle contractions while the parasympathetic stimulation decreases the rate and force of contraction.

17. _____ Sympathetic stimulation of the autonomic system decreases activity of visceral smooth muscles, whereas parasympathetic stimulation increases these muscles.

18. _____ As with visceral muscle cells, multiunit smooth muscle cells are linked as a unit to the autonomic nervous system.

19. _____ Loose and dense connective tissue both have fiber-producing cells, fibroblasts, and three types of fibers—collagen fibers, reticular fibers, and elastic fibers.

20. _____ The pelvis is composed of the ileum, the ischium, and the pubis.

21. _____ The patella is the largest sesamoid bone in the body.

22. _____ The bones of the visceral skeleton include the os penis, os cordis, and os rostri.

23. _____ Fibrous joints are movable, cartilaginous joints are slightly movable, and diarthrodial or synovial joints are immovable.

24. _____ Adipose connective tissue, or fat, consists of collections of lipid-storing cells.

25. _____ Subcutaneous injections are administered in the hypodermis layer of loose connective tissue.

PLACE IN ORDER

Order the items below from distal to proximal.

1. _____   A. Tarsus
                  B. Femur
2. _____   C. Metatarsus
                  D. Pelvis
3. _____   E. Tibia/fibula
                  F. Patella
4. _____   G. Phalanges
5. _____

6. _____

7. _____

FILL IN THE BLANK

1. The six main types of connective tissues present in the body are:

   a. _____

   b. _____

   c. _____

   d. _____

   e. _____

   f. _____

2. Six potential joint movements in the body are:

a. _____

b. _____

c. _____

d. _____

e. _____

f. _____

3. Purposes of the integument include:

a. _____

b. _____

c. _____

d. _____

e. _____

PHOTO QUIZ

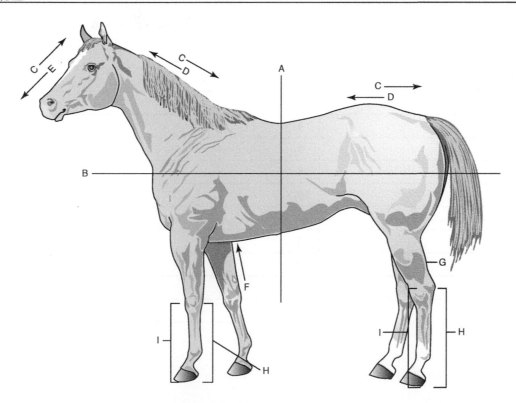

Label the letters according to the terms denoting position in animals.

A.	B.
C.	D.
E.	F.
G.	H.
I.	J.

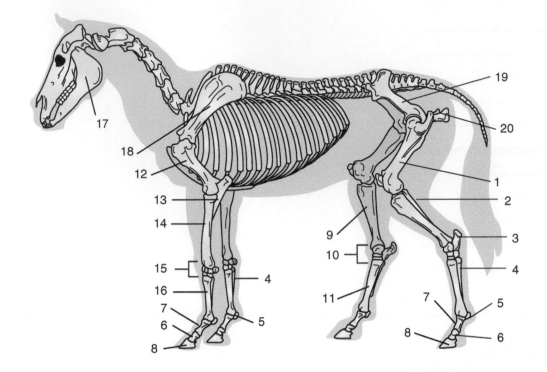

Label the numbered anatomic parts of the horse.

1.	2.
3.	4.
5.	6.
7.	8.
9.	10.
11.	12.
13.	14.
15.	16.
17.	18.
19.	20.

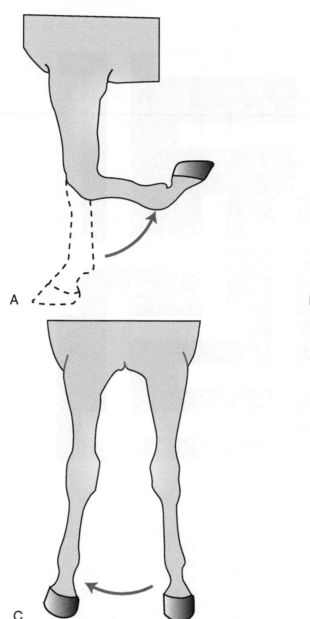
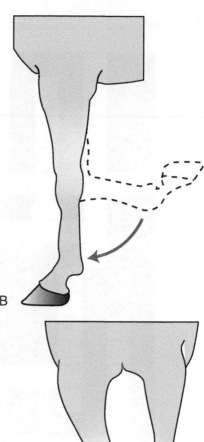

The arrows in each case represent which direction?

A.	
B.	
C.	
D.	

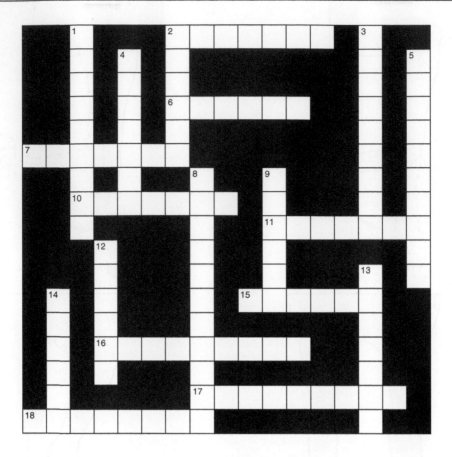

Across

2 Pertaining to the head end of the body. (7)
6 Farther from the center of the body, relative to another body part. (6)
7 Toward the nose. (7)
10 At an angle. (7)
11 Pertaining to the undersurface of the rear foot. (7)
15 Denoting a position closer to the median plane of a body, relative to another body part. (6)
16 Movement of a limb or part away from the median line. (9)
17 Movement of a limb or part toward the median line. (9)
18 Nearer to the center of the body, relative to another body part. (8)

Down

1 The act of straightening a joint. (9)
2 Pertaining to the tail end of the body. (6)
3 Lying down. (9)
4 Pertaining to the underside of a quadruped. (7)
5 Situated near the outermost part or surface of an organ or body part. (10)
8 Situation near the surface of the body; the opposite of "deep." (11)
9 Lying face up. (6)
12 Pertaining to the back area of a quadruped. (6)
13 The act of bending a joint. (7)
14 Pertaining to the undersurface of the front foot. (6)

6 Diagnostic Imaging

LEARNING OBJECTIVES

After reviewing this chapter, the reader will be able to:
- Describe the components of the x-ray machine and the function of each part
- Explain how x-rays are produced
- Discuss the factors that affect radiographic quality
- Describe techniques and devices used to optimize radiographic quality
- Discuss the dangers of radiation and methods to avoid radiation injury
- Describe the procedures used to develop radiographs
- Explain proper positioning of animals for various radiographic studies
- Describe the basic physics of ultrasound
- List the components of ultrasound machines and the function of each part
- List the non–x-ray imaging modalities and provide an overview of each.

LABEL

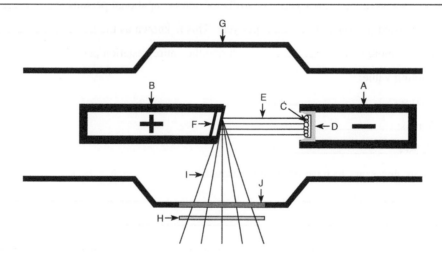

Identify the elements in the illustration.

A. _____

B. _____

C. _____

D. _____

E. _____

F. _____

G. _____

H. _____

I. _____

J. _____

1. Radiographs that show a (**long/short**) scale of contrast have a few black and white shades, with (**a few/many**) shades of gray. A (**long/short**) scale of contrast has black-and-white shades, with (**a few/many**) shades of gray in between. For most studies, a (**short/long**) scale of contrast is desirable.

2. What four factors must be considered to obtain the proper scale of radiographic contrast:

   a. _____

   b. _____

   c. _____

   d. _____

3. Denser tissues, such as bone, absorb (**greater/less**) amounts of x-rays and appear (**white/black**) on a radiograph while less dense tissues, such as lung tissue, absorb (**greater/less**) x-rays and appear (**white/black**) on the finished radiograph

4. As kVp (**increases/decreases**), the scale of contrast gets longer and there is (**more/less**) exposure latitude which is forgiving of minor technique errors.

5. The National Council on Radiation Protection and Measurements recommends that the dose for occupationally exposed persons not exceed _____ per year The MPD for non-occupational persons is _____ for occupationally exposed persons, or _____ per year. This is known as the _____. Also, a fetus should not receive more than _____ during the entire gestation period.

6. Calculate the remaining value:

   a. 100 mA and 1/20 sec: _____ mas

   b. 300 mA and 5 mAs: _____ sec

   c. 10 mAs and 1/25sec: _____ mA

7. What preparations are necessary to have optimal ultrasound?

   a. _____

   b. _____

   c. _____

   d. _____

   e. _____

8. What procedures are required to prepare for endoscopy?

   a. _____

   b. _____

   c. _____

   d. _____

   e. _____

   f. _____

   g. _____

   h. _____

   i. _____

   j. _____

9. Explain some procedures involved with the care of endoscopes:

   a. _____

   b. _____

   c. _____

   d. _____

   e. _____

   f. _____

   g. _____

   h. _____

   i. _____

   j. _____

   k. _____

10. Describe some checks that can be completed if proper brightness cannot be achieved when performing an ultrasound.

   a. _____

   b. _____

   c. _____

   d. _____

   e. _____

11. List important safety rules that should be kept in mind while radiographing.

   a. _____

   b. _____

   c. _____

   d. _____

   e. _____

   f. _____

   g. _____

   h. _____

12. To INCREASE radiographic density you must do what to the following?

A. mAs	1) Increase	2) Decrease	3) Does not affect
B. kVp	1) Increase	2) Decrease	3) Does not affect
C. Tissue density	1) Increase	2) Decrease	3) Does not affect
D. Tissue thickness	1) Increase	2) Decrease	3) Does not affect
E. Atomic number of object	1) Increase	2) Decrease	3) Does not affect
F. Source image distance	1) Farther away	2) Closer	3) Does not affect
G. Temperature of processing solutions	1) Increase	2) Decrease	3) Does not affect
H. Grid use	1) No grid	2) Use a grid	3) Does not affect
I. Foreshortening	1) Increase	2) Decrease	3) Does not affect
J. Film speed	1) Increase	2) Decrease	3) Does not affect
K. Screen speed	1) Increase	2) Decrease	3) Does not affect

13. To INCREASE radiographic contrast you must do what to the following?

A. mAs	1) Increase	2) Decrease	3) Does not affect
B. kVp	1) Increase	2) Decrease	3) Does not affect
C. Tissue density	1) Increase	2) Decrease	3) Does not affect
D. Atomic number of object	1) Increase	2) Decrease	3) Does not affect
E. Source image distance	1) Farther away	2) Closer	3) Does not affect
F. Temperature of processing solutions	1) Increase	2) Decrease	3) Does not affect
G. Grid use	1) Use	2) Do not use	3) Does not affect
H. Foreshortening	1) Increase	2) Decrease	3) Does not affect
I. Focal spot size	1) Increase	2) Decrease	3) Does not affect
J. Contrast scale	1) Longer	2) Shorter	3) Does not affect
K. Fogging	1) Increase	2) Decrease	3) Does not affect
L. Use of collimator	1) Use	2) Do not use	3) Does not affect
M. Use of filter	1) Use	2) Do not use	3) Does not affect
N. Use of Potter-Bucky	1) Use	2) Do not use	3) Does not affect

14. To INCREASE radiographic detail you must do what to the following?

A. mAs   1) Increase   2) Decrease   3) Does not affect

B. kVp   1) Increase   2) Decrease   3) Does not affect

C. Focal spot size   1) Increase   2) Decrease   3) Does not affect

D. Source image distance   1) Farther away   2) Closer   3) Does not affect

E. Object image distance   1) Farther away   2) Closer   3) Does not affect

F. Temperature of processing solutions   1) Increase   2) Decrease   3) Does not affect

G. Foreshortening   1) Parallel   2) Angled   3) Does not affect

H. Film speed   1) Increase   2) Decrease   3) Does not affect

I. Screen speed   1) Increase   2) Decrease   3) Does not affect

15. Fill in the meanings of the acronyms:

1. REM   _____

2. SV   _____

3. rad   _____

4. GY   _____

5. ALARA   _____

6. MPD   _____

7. NCRPM   _____

16. Fill in the following chart:

Body Part	Cranial or Proximal Landmark	Caudal or Distal Landmark	Center Landmark	Comments
Abdomen				Take at peak _____
Thorax				Take at peak _____
Pelvis			✕	✕
Stifle				✕
Radius/ulna				✕
Lumbar vertebrae			✕	To increase detail _____

Place the following sequence of events of manual processing in order.

_____ 1.

_____ 2.

_____ 3.

_____ 4.

_____ 5.

_____ 6.

_____ 7.

_____ 8.

_____ 9.

_____ 10.

_____ 11.

_____ 12.

A. Lift the film out of the wash tank, allowing the excess water to drain back into wash tank.

B. Place the film into the fixer tank for the appropriate time and agitate gently to dislodge air bubbles that cling to the surface.

C. After washing the film, let it hang until dry.

D. Place the film in the wash tank for at least 30 minutes.

E. Turn on water to the wash tank.

F. Immerse the film in the developer.

G. Unload the cassette and place the film on the appropriate size film hanger.

H. After proper developing time, place the film in the wash tank and agitate for 30 seconds.

I. Gently agitate the film to dislodge any air bubbles that may cling to the film's surface.

J. Check chemical levels and stir both chemical tanks.

K. Turn on the safelight and turn off the white lights.

L. Check chemical temperature.

Match the key terms associated with radiographic quality.

_____ 1. Anode heel effect

_____ 2. Radiographic density

_____ 3. Radiographic contrast

_____ 4. Subject density

_____ 5. Radiographic detail

_____ 6. Artifacts

_____ 7. Penumbra

A. Loss of detail due to geometric unsharpness

B. Unwanted density in the form of blemishes

C. The sharp interfaces between tissues and organs

D. Unequal distribution of the x-ray beam intensity

E. Differences in radiographic density between adjacent areas on a radiographic image

F. Degree of blackness on a radiograph

G. The ability of the different tissue densities to absorb x-rays

Match the terms associated with processing.

_____ 1. Acidifier

_____ 2. Activator

_____ 3. Fixing agent

_____ 4. Hardener

_____ 5. Main purpose of the developer

_____ 6. Main purpose of the fixer

_____ 7. Preservative

_____ 8. Reducing agent

_____ 9. Restrainer

_____ 10. Solvent

A. Causes film emulsion to swell

B. Found in both solutions; sodium or potassium sulfite is used

C. Prevents the reducing agents from affecting the unsensitized crystals

D. Provides an alkaline pH in the range of 9.8 to 11.4

E. Hardens and prevents excessive swelling of the film emulsion

F. Neutralizes any alkaline developer remaining on the film

G. Clears the unchanged silver halide crystals from the film emulsion, leaving the black metallic silver

H. Change the sensitized silver halide crystals into black metallic silver

I. Convert the exposed silver halide crystals to black metallic silver

J. The sodium or ammonium thiosulfate that clears the remaining silver halide crystals in the fixer

Match the terms associated with positioning.

_____ 1. Ventral (V):

_____ 2. Dorsal (D):

_____ 3. Medial (M):

_____ 4. Lateral (L):

_____ 5. Cranial (Cr):

_____ 6. Caudal (Cd):

_____ 7. Rostral (R):

_____ 8. Palmar (Pa):

_____ 9. Plantar (Pl):

_____ 10. Proximal (Pr):

_____ 11. Distal (Di):

A. Situated closer to the point of attachment or origin

B. Situated on the caudal aspect of the rear limb, distal to the tarsus

C. Areas on the head situated toward the nose
D. Body area situated toward the median plane or midline
E. Situated away from the point of attachment or origin
F. Structures or areas situated toward the head
G. Body area situated toward the underside of quadrupeds
H. Structures or areas situated toward the tail
I. Situated on the caudal aspect of the front limb, distal to the carpus
J. Body area situated toward the back or topline of quadrupeds
K. Body area situated away from the median plane or midline

Match the terms associated with alternate imaging.

_____ 1. A-mode

_____ 2. B-mode

_____ 3. M-mode

_____ 4. Echogenic

_____ 5. Sonolucent

_____ 6. Anechoic

_____ 7. Hyperechoic

_____ 8. Hypoechoic

_____ 9. Isoechoic

_____ 10. Gain and power

_____ 11. Total gain compensation

_____ 12. Near field gain and far field gain

_____ 13. Acoustic shadowing

_____ 14. Distance enhancement

_____ 15. Slice thickness

_____ 16. Reverberation

_____ 17. Mirror-image

_____ 18. CT scanner

_____ 19. MRI

A. Returning echoes displayed as bright pixels or dots on a screen
B. Continuous display of a thin slice of an organ over time
C. Returning echoes displayed as a series of peaks on a graph
D. Sound is transmitted to the deeper tissues, appearing dark on the screen
E. Sound is reflected back to the transducer, appearing white on the screen
F. Tissues that reflect more sound back to the transducer than surrounding tissues so they appear brighter than surrounding tissues
G. Tissue that appears to have the same echotexture on the screen as surrounding tissues
H. No sound reflected back to the transducer, appearing black on the screen
I. Tissues that reflect less sound back to the transducer than surrounding tissues so they appear darker than surrounding tissues
J. Part of TGC that controls the amount of electronic gain added to the sound returning from the near field or far field, respectively
K. Occurs when the sound beam traverses a cystic structure so that tissues deep to the cystic structure appear brighter than surrounding tissues
L. A series of lines an equal distance apart on the screen that occurs when sound is reflected off a highly reflective interface and then reflected back into the tissues by the surface of the transducer
M. An artifact that occurs when imaging an anechoic or hypoechoic structure
N. Affects the overall brightness of the image and compensates for attenuation of the sound beam as it travels through the tissues
O. Occurs when the sound is attenuated or reflected at an acoustic interface, preventing the sound from being transmitted to the deeper tissues
P. An artefact common when viewing the liver and diaphragm
Q. The purpose is to make like tissues look alike
R. Use of high-strength external magnetic field, radiofrequency excitation pulses, and natural resonance of protons
S. A cross-sectional image of all tissue types of the body region scanned based on the physical density of the tissue compared to water

1. What are the agents along with the solvent that are in the fixer:
   a. reducing agent, fixing agent, accelerator, and acidifier
   b. clearing agent, preservative, hardener, acidifier, and buffer
   c. reducing agent, accelerator, preservative, restrainer, and hardener
   d. buffer, accelerator, acidifier, clearing agent, and hardener

2. With manual processing using the exhaustion method, the solution that is going to be diluted the most is the:
   a. developer
   b. fixer
   c. both will be diluted equally

3. The temperature of your manual developer is 65° F (18° C). If you were to process at this temperature, your time should be:
   a. 3¾ minutes
   b. 5¾ minutes
   c. 6¼ minutes
   d. 7½ minutes

4. You are doing a safelight quality control test with an initial moderate exposure. There is no area of increased density. This means that:
   a. There is no problem with the safelight or light leaking around the door.
   b. You need to get a brand new safelight; otherwise, you will always have fogging.
   c. You have less than 30 seconds to get the film into the processing solutions.
   d. You must have completed the test incorrectly.

5. There is an interesting correlation between kVp and electromagnetic radiation. Generally as the:
   a. kVp is increased, the penetration is increased
   b. kVp is increased, the penetration is decreased
   c. kVp is decreased, the penetration is increased
   d. kVp is decreased, the penetration is decreased

6. Which one of the following statements regarding the production of x-rays is false?
   a. The target and focal spot are provided by the anode.
   b. The cathode side of the tube is positive and the anode is negative.
   c. The cathode provides the focusing cup, filament, and method of acceleration.
   d. The vacuum environment is provided by the glass envelope.

7. Which of the following lists has objects ordered from least subject density to most subject density?
   a. metal, bone, water, fat, and gas
   b. fat, water, gas, bone and metal
   c. water, gas, fat, bone and metal
   d. gas, fat, water, bone and metal

8. With regards to radiation exposure of pregnant women and those under 18:
   a. Technically the law states that there is no more concern for these women than for others who are occupationally exposed.
   b. The law states that they should never be in the room during the exposure.
   c. The dermis, bone, and blood cells are the most sensitive to ionizing radiation.
   d. The growth and gonadal cells are most sensitive to ionizing radiation.

9. The quality of the beam refers to:
   a. kVp
   b. mAs
   c. rectification that is required
   d. darkness of the radiograph

10. Scatter will be more noticeable if there is a thicker patient and:
    a. lower kVp and larger field size
    b. lower kVp and smaller field size
    c. higher kVp and smaller field size
    d. higher kVp and larger field size

11. When you change the mAs from 5 to 10, you are:
    a. decreasing both radiographic contrast and radiographic density
    b. increasing both radiographic contrast and radiographic density
    c. increasing radiographic contrast and decreasing radiographic density
    d. not changing the radiographic contrast but increasing the radiographic density

12. Bone as compared to a kidney will have:
    a. less radiographic contrast and less radiographic density
    b. less radiographic contrast and greater radiographic density
    c. greater radiographic contrast and less radiographic density
    d. greater radiographic contrast and greater radiographic density

13. A radiograph has light image density. To improve the image:
    a. increase either the kVp or mAs
    b. decrease either the kVp or mAs
    c. increase the source image distance
    d. use a grid

14. If the source image distance is changed from 100 cm to 50 cm, what will the new mAs be if the old mAs was 24?
    a. 48
    b. 24
    c. 12
    d. 6

15. A film has low contrast when there are:
    a. blacks and whites with a short scale
    b. blacks and whites with a long scale
    c. grays with a long scale
    d. grays with a short scale

16. The same exposure was taken in two radiographs but the grid had been used for one. The one using the grid would be the:
    a. darker radiograph
    b. lighter radiograph

17. Compared to a fast screen, a slow screen will:
    a. have greater detail, less graininess, and more latitude and require more mAs
    b. have greater detail, more graininess, and more latitude and require more mAs
    c. have less detail, more graininess, and more latitude and require more mAs
    d. have less detail, more graininess, and less latitude and require less mAs

18. The rare earth screens emit which color of light when they fluoresce?
    a. green
    b. blue
    c. clear
    d. mauve

19. Why, in spite of the decreased SID, do teeth not appear blurry or show poor detail when radiographs are taken at the dentist?
    a. as SID decreases the detail increases.
    b. nonscreen film requires many fewer exposure factors, so there is less chance of movement.
    c. nonscreen film is exposed by direct radiation, not by the light emitted from screens.
    d. there is more quantum mottle with direct film,

20. As the mAs is increased:
    a. contrast is decreased
    b. contrast is increased
    c. contrast is not changed, because mAs does not affect contrast

21. As the kVp is increased:
    a. contrast is decreased
    b. contrast is increased
    c. contrast is not changed, because kVp does not affect contrast

22. The SID has decreased as you take dental radiographs. The image will now appear:
    a. larger
    b. smaller
    c. the same size, because SID does not affect this.

23. When the small focal spot is used, the edges of the image will appear:
    a. sharper
    b. not as detailed

24. Which of the following is a positive contrast medium that draws fluid into the GI?
    a. air
    b. barium sulphate
    c. ionic water-soluble organic iodides

25. Which of the following is a contrast agent that can be injected into the vascular system?
    a. air
    b. barium sulphate
    c. ionic water-soluble organic iodides

26. Which of the following is a positive contrast used when there is a perforation in the bowel?
    a. air
    b. barium sulphate
    c. ionic water-soluble organic iodides

27. Which of the following is a positive contrast medium that becomes diluted?
    a. air
    b. barium sulphate
    c. ionic water-soluble organic iodides

28. Which of the following is a radiolucent substance?
    a. air
    b. barium sulphate
    c. ionic water-soluble organic iodides

29. Which of the following is a contrast medium that remains inert in a body cavity?
    a. air
    b. barium sulphate
    c. ionic water-soluble organic iodides

30. Which of the following is the most appropriate contrast medium for positive contrast cystography in dogs?
    a. air
    b. barium sulphate
    c. ionic water-soluble organic iodides

31. Which of the following is a best used for myelography?
    a. air
    b. barium sulphate
    c. ionic water-soluble organic iodides
    d. nonionic water-soluble organic iodides are used for myelography

32. Which agent has the lowest atomic number?
    a. air
    b. barium sulphate
    c. ionic water-soluble organic iodides
    d. nonionic water-soluble organic iodides are used for myelography

33. When utilizing endoscopes:
    a. Use the rigid endoscopes for GI studies or female cystoscopy.
    b. Flexible endoscopes are best used for laparoscopy or rhinoscopy.
    c. Hold the rigid endoscope by the rod.
    d. Fiberoptic endoscopes use glass fiber bundles for transmission of images.

34. If involved with MRI, it is important to keep in mind that:
    a. Latex gloves or lab coats are not needed if handling radionuclide or a radioactive patient.
    b. There is no excretion of radionuclides in urine and feces.
    c. Isolation or a well-ventilated area is not required if radionuclides are injected.
    d. An anesthetic machine could cause serious damage to the MRI machine.

35. For digital radiography:
    a. DR system has an imaging plate that stores the radiation received, taking the place of a cassette.
    b. CR system has an imaging plate comprised of detectors connected directly to the computer.
    c. CCD system requires a new radiology generator and table
    d. The CR system is the most expensive.

TRUE OR FALSE

1. _____ Penumbra can be minimized by increasing the size of the focal spot.

2. _____ Increasing the kVp increases the scatter produced.

3. _____ If you use 16 mAs at 40 inches (100 cm) SID, the mAs is 4 at a SID of 20 inches (50 cm).

4. _____ As you increase the object image distance, you are decreasing penumbra.

5. _____ If the limb is not parallel to the film, you may have foreshortening.

6. _____ The collimator in an x-ray tube head focuses the primary beam to a narrower image.

7. _____ For safety reasons, it best to use a lower mA but a longer time.

8. _____ The higher the mA setting on the x-ray machine, the greater the number of x-rays produced. The higher the kVp, the greater the penetrating power of the x-rays.

9. _____ Keeping all other factors constant and changing the mAs from 5 to 10 will double the radiographic density.

10. _____ Changing the SID does not affect the penetrating power of the beam, so kVp remains constant.

11. _____ If there was no image on a film that was exposed to radiation and it was processed normally, the film would appear black.

12. _____ Light leak around one edge of the film will appear white.

13. _____ Thumbnail pressure on a film after exposure but before processing will show as a crescent black mark.

14. _____ A hair on the film during exposure to radiation will appear black.

15. _____ Rare earth phosphors are the most common blue light–emitting phosphors.

16. _____ Film with long or increased latitude can produce images with a long scale of contrast (many shades of gray).

17. _____ Digital radiography includes computed radiography (CR), digital radiography (DR), and coupled charged device (CCD) technologies.

18. _____ For CCD digital radiography, imaging plate (IP) contains a photostimulable phosphor.

19. _____ Digital radiographs, CT, MRI, and ultrasound images are all stored using a universally accepted format known as DICOM.

20. _____ A PACS has the advantage of storing multiple patients and making images available to multiple computers within a hospital or a network of hospitals.

21. _____ Radiation cannot penetrate lead gloves and thus cause any ionization of intracellular water that releases toxic products, which can damage the DNA.

22. _____ Effects may be somatic or carcinogenic when radiation comes in contact with the cells of living tissue, either passing through the cells with no effect, producing cell damage that is repairable or not repairable, or killing the cells.

23. _____ Tissues that are most sensitive to ionizing radiation are those with rapidly growing or reproducing cells, including lymphocytic series, reproductive, GI, or lens of the eye.

24. _____ Intrauterine lethality is most critical from 0 to 9 days, while the period of organogenesis (10 days to 6 weeks) carries the greatest risk of congenital malformation in the fetus.

25. _____ Radiograph lead gloves and lead gowns at 5 mAs and 80 kVp every 18 months.

26. _____ The most important feature of a darkroom is that it must be light tight.

27. _____ X-rays must be labeled with the clinic name and location, date the x-ray was taken, owner's name, and, patient's name.

28. _____ A red lightbulb can substitute as a safelight filter.

29. _____ The safelight that is effective against blue light–sensitive film can also be used with greenlight–sensitive film.

30. _____ If either the replenishing method or the exhausted method is used for manual processing, the chemicals should be changed every 3 months.

31. _____ In automatic processors, the chemicals are kept at temperatures around 80° F (27° C).

32. _____ Label the radiograph of the oblique so that a marker is placed to indicate the direction of entry and exit of the primary beam.

33. _____ In an ultrasound, soft tissues are represented as many shades of gray.

34. _____ Structures that can cause acoustic shadowing include bone, calculi, mineralized tissues, and fat, and the shadowing is more pronounced with lower-frequency transducers.

35. _____ The controls that make up the time gain compensation (TGC) are the most important and most often improperly set.

36. _____ All artefacts during ultrasound are an inconvenience, especially acoustic shadowing and distance enhancement.

37. _____ It is essential during endoscopy that the endotracheal tube cuff remain uninflated while extubating.

38. _____ Depending on the MRI scan performed, a contrast medium such as gadolinium may or may not be administered to brighten tissues such as vessels and tumors.

39. _____ Microchips can cause serious damage to an MRI machine.

40. _____ Another term for nuclear medicine is scintigraphy, an imaging modality that utilizes radionuclides.

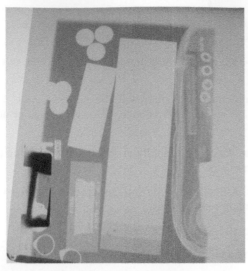

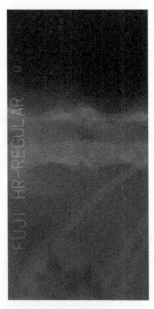

1. Why does the radiograph show a low density?

_____

_____

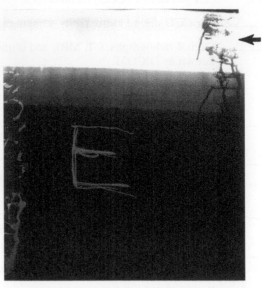

2. This film was exposed to light and then processed. Why would there be a clear area at the upper portion of the film? What has caused the blackened area under the arrow.

_____

_____

3. This is considered a **(low/high)**-contrast film.

_____

_____

4. Has this film been exposed to radiation? What are the darkened areas at the edges due to?

_____

_____

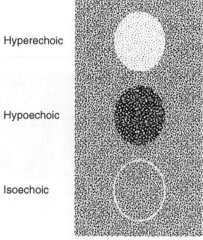

Hyperechoic

Hypoechoic

Isoechoic

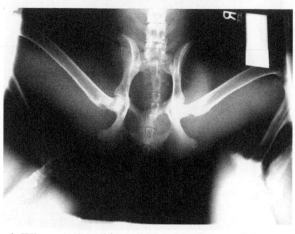

5. From upper to lower, what are the three ultrasound areas shown in the circled areas?

_____

_____

6. What are the white areas at the corners of the radiograph and why is this a problem?

_____

_____

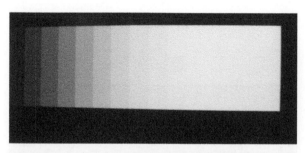

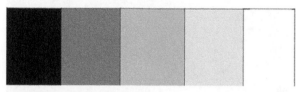

7. The whitest area is the (**thickest/thinnest**) portion of the step wedge.

_____

_____

8. From left to right, what tissue densities are represented with each area?

_____

_____

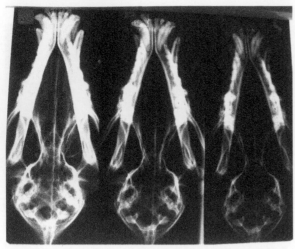

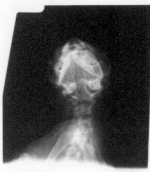

9. The skull on the left is larger because of **(increased/decreased)** OFD. Assuming that there has been a corresponding change in exposure factors, the skull on the left could also be larger because of **(shorter/longer)** SID.

_____

_____

10. The skull on the left has **(lower/higher)** kVP and is considered to have **(lower/higher)** contrast.

_____

_____

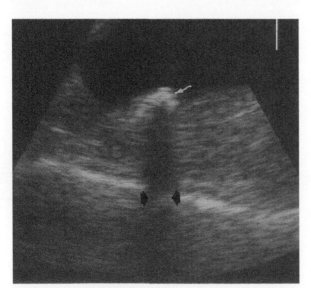

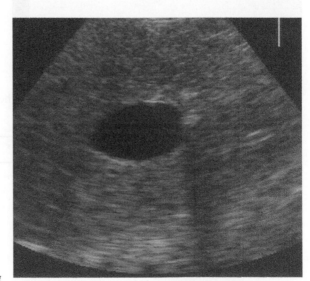

11. What artifact is shown? The white arrow is pointing to the _____ while the black arrowheads are pointing to the _____.

_____

_____

12. What is this US artifact due to?

_____

_____

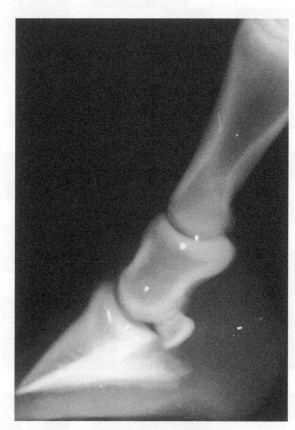

13. What has caused the white artifacts?

_____

_____

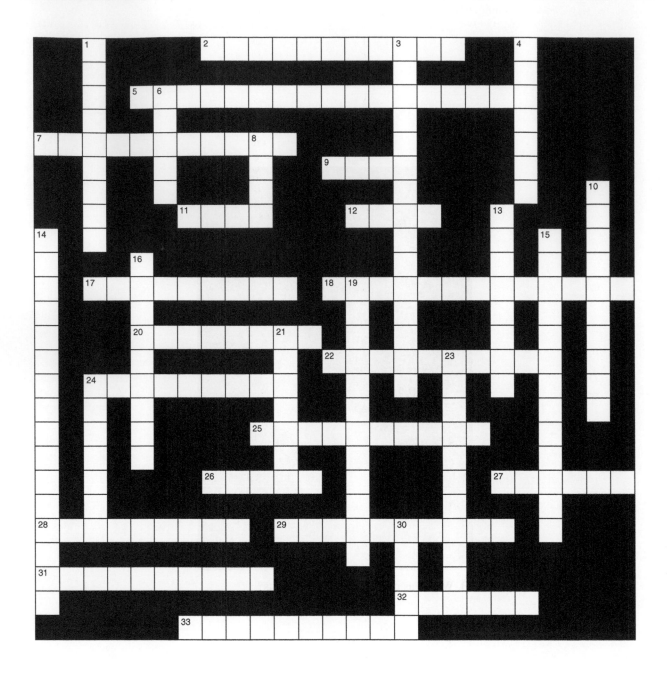

Across

2 An imaging technique using contrast media to visualize the spinal cord. (11)

5 MRI, or ___ ___ imaging, is a modality that utilizes a magnetic field that recognizes the natural resonance of the atoms within the body to produce images. (2 words) (17)

7 The ___ peak is the voltage applied across an x-ray tube that determines the energy of the electrons produced. (11)

9 The acronym for dedicated computer systems used for storing, retrieving, transferring, and manipulating images. (4)

11 One form of electromagnetic radiation. (4)

12 A ___ is a device that is made up of lead strips interspaced with a radiolucent material. It absorbs scatter radiation. (4)

17 Substances that emit light when exposed to electromagnetic radiation. (9)

18 The current produced by the x-ray tube during an exposure. (13)

20 A structure not normally present but visible on a radiograph. It diminishes the quality of the radiograph. (8)

22 An example of when there is greater radiation intensity on the negatively charged side of an x-ray tube due to the angle of the target on the positively charged side. (2 words) (10)

24 A low wattage light bulb and special filter that will not affect radiographic film. (9)

25 A device on an x-ray machine that consists of lead plates and is used to reduce scatter radiation. (10)

26 A chemical solution that clears unchanged silver halide crystals on an exposed x-ray film. (5)

27 The ___ image is the invisible image that is within the emulsion of an x-ray film produced after the film has been exposed to light. (6)

28 ___ elements are photosensitive elements such as lanthanum oxybromide and gadolinium oxysulfide that are in an x-ray–intensifying screen. (2 words) (9)

29 The device on an ultrasound machine that emits and receives a sound wave signal that converts the waves into electrical impulses. (10)

31 Ultrasound is a modality that utilizes ___ ___ that interact with tissue interfaces and are reflected back to create an image. (2 words) (10)

32 Negative contrast agents are gases such as ___ and carbon dioxide that are radiolucent on radiographs that are used to outline organs. (6)

33 The ___ distance is the distance between the object being radiographed and the film or plate. (2 words) (10)

Down

1 A chemical solution that converts exposed silver halide crystals to black metallic silver. (9)

3 Being able to store a latent image that may be freed as light when stimulated by a scanning laser. (15)

4 The dose of radiation equivalent to the absorbed dose by tissue. (7)

6 The positively charged electrode in an x-ray tube. (5)

8 The measured unit of radiation dose that is absorbed due to ionized radiation. (4)

10 CT, or computed ___, is a modality that utilizes an x-ray tube that freely rotates around a patient, creating a dataset of images. (10)

13 ___ radiography is a type of digital radiography that utilizes a cassette screen system. (8)

14 A type of medium such as barium or iodine that is radiopaque on radiographs used to visualize organs in the body. (2 words) (16)

15 ___ ___ radiography is a type of digital radiography that utilizes an imaging plate of detectors connected directly to a computer system. (2 words) (13)

16 The ___ distance is the distance that is measured from the target of the x-ray tube to the radiographic film or plate. (2 words) (9)

19 ___ screens are plates within the x-ray cassette that are comprised of phosphorescent crystals that function to emit light. (12)

21 The negatively charged electrode in an x-ray tube that produces electrons. (7)

23 An imaging technique that produces a continual stream of images. (11)

24 ___ radiation is the radiation created as a result of the interaction of primary beam x-ray photons and body parts or matter that travel in a different direction and are composed of lower energies. (7)

30 The acronym for the universal method in which medical imaging can be stored and transferred. (5)

7 Hematology and Hemostasis

LEARNING OBJECTIVES

After reviewing this chapter, the reader will be able to:
- Describe methods used to collect blood samples for laboratory examination
- Describe preparation of diagnostic samples for laboratory examination
- List and describe common procedures used for hematologic examinations
- Describe characteristics of normal and common abnormal cells in peripheral blood
- Discuss methods used to maintain accuracy of laboratory test results
- List and describe methods for evaluation of hemostasis in domestic animals

DEFINITIONS

Define the following terms:

1. Absolute value _____

2. Anemia _____

3. Heterophil _____

4. Left shift _____

5. Lipemia _____

6. Poikilocytosis _____

7. Rouleaux _____

8. Polycythemia _____

9. Pancytopenia _____

10. Polychromasia _____

MATCHING

Match the following cells with their functions:

1. _____ Neutrophil

2. _____ Eosinophil

3. _____ Basophil

4. _____ Monocyte

5. _____ Lymphocyte

A. Allergic reactions, phagocytosis
B. Precursors to tissue macrophage; phagocytosis and processing of antigens
C. Phagocytosis and destruction of foreign agents and cellular debris
D. Cytokine production and cell-mediated immune response; antibody production
E. Initiation and mediation of immune responses and hypersensitivity allergic reactions

SHORT ANSWER

1. Differentiate between accuracy and precision.

_____

_____

_____

_____

2. List the cells in the granulocyte maturation series in order from most immature to most mature.

_____

_____

_____

3. List five common clinical signs of hemostatic defects.

_____

_____

_____

4. List the equations used for calculation of erythrocyte indices.

_____

_____

_____

_____

_____

_____

5. Describe the procedure for performing the PCV by the microhematocrit method.

_____

_____

_____

_____

_____

_____

_____

_____

TRUE OR FALSE

_____ 1. Samples for hematology testing should be collected from a properly fasted animal.

_____ 2. The cephalic vein is the preferred site for blood collection in all dogs and cats.

_____ 3. Heparin is the preferred anticoagulant for hematology testing.

_____ 4. Sodium citrate anticoagulant is used for coagulation tests.

_____ 5. Impedance analyzers quantify cells in a sample based on their size and density

_____ 6. Neutrophils are the most common leukocyte found in the blood of most mammals.

_____ 7. The most common inherited coagulation disorder of domestic animals is vonWillebrand disease

_____ 8. The most common secondary coagulation disorders of domestic animals results from Ehrlichiosis.

_____ 9. The prothrombin time test is used to evaluate the intrinsic coagulation pathway.

_____ 10. The D-Dimer test can be used to evaluate tertiary hemostasis.

Identify the term described and unscramble the letters in parentheses to reveal the hidden word:

1. Decrease in circulating platelets

2. The granulocyte stem cell

3. The erythrocyte stem cell

4. The largest leukocyte found in the peripheral blood of most mammals

5. The term for pinpoint hemorrhage

6. Decrease in the oxygen-carrying ability of the blood

7. An infectious agent of RBCs that appears as a large, round, oval, or teardrop-shaped body

8. The bone marrow cell that gives rise to thrombocytes

9. Variation in cell size

10. Type of reticulocyte unique to cats

11. Red blood cells with long, irregular surface projections

Super Clue

Fragmented erythrocytes usually formed as a result of shearing of the red cell by intravascular trauma

1. __ __ __ __ __ __ __ __ __ __ __ __ (__) __ __ __

2. __ __ __ __ __ __ __ __ (__) __

3. __ __ __ __ (__) __ __ __ __ __ __ __

4. __ __ __ __ __ __ (__) __

5. __ __ __ __ __ (__) __ __

6. __ __ __ __ (__) __

7. __ __ __ __ (__) __ __

8. __ __ __ __ __ __ __ __ (__) __ __ __ __

9. __ __ __ __ __ (__) __ __ __ __

10. __ __ __ __ (__) __ __ __ __ __

11. __ __ __ (__) __ __ __ __

Super Clue __ __ __ __ __ __ __ __ __ __

Match the terms below with the photos on the right.

_____ 1. Schistocytes

A.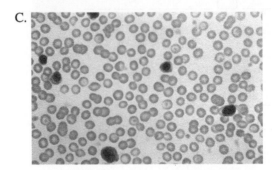

_____ 2. Echinocytes

B.

_____ 3. Hypochromasia

C.

_____ 4. Rouleaux

D.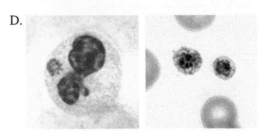

_____ 5. Heinz Bodies

E.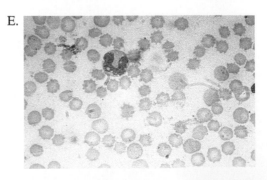

_____ 6. Nucleated red blood cells

F.

_____ 7. *Mycoplasma felis*

G.

_____ 8. *Ehrlichia*

H.

_____ 9. Lymphocytes

I.

_____ 10. Monocytes

J.

_____ 11. Hypersegmentation   K.

_____ 12. Toxic neutrophils with Döhle bodies   L.

SHORT ANSWER

1. List six possible causes and solutions for excessive blue coloration on stained slides:

    1. _____

    2. _____

    3. _____

    4. _____

    5. _____

    6. _____

2. List six possible causes and solutions for excessive pink coloration on stained slides:

    1. _____

    2. _____

    3. _____

    4. _____

    5. _____

    6. _____

3. Describe the procedure for performing a platelet estimate:

    _____

    _____

    _____

    _____

4. Describe the procedure for performing a reticulocyte count:

_____

_____

_____

_____

5. Describe the manual method for performing fibrinogen determination:

_____

_____

_____

_____

WORD SEARCH

Identify the term described and then find the terms in the Word Search.

1. Abnormal decrease in neutrophils in a peripheral blood sample _____

2. Abnormal increase in neutrophils in a peripheral blood sample _____

3. Abnormal yellowish discoloration of skin, mucous membranes, or plasma as a result of increased concentration of bile pigments _____

4. An anuclear, immature erythrocyte _____

5. An increase in the numbers of circulating erythrocytes _____

6. Any abnormal cell shape _____

7. Arrangement of erythrocytes in a column or stack _____

8. Blood coagulation _____

9. Bluish-gray appearance of cells or components of cells that have high affinity for stains with alkaline pH

_____

10. Bone marrow cell from which blood platelets arise _____

11. Cells that appear with their characteristic morphology _____

12. Cells that stain with their characteristic color _____

13. Decrease in circulating platelets _____

14. Decreased number of leukocytes in blood _____

15. Decreased numbers of all blood cells and platelets in a peripheral blood or bone marrow sample

_____

16. Denotes a neutrophil with more than five nuclear lobes _____

17. Destruction of erythrocytes _____

18. Erythrocytes with decreased staining intensity due to decrease in hemoglobin concentration

_____

19. Fragmented erythrocytes usually formed as a result of shearing of the red cell by intravascular trauma

_____

20. Immature granulocyte with parallel sides and no nuclear lobed or indentations _____

21. Increased numbers of leukocytes in the blood _____

22. Instrument used to measure the refractive index of a solution _____

23. Layer of material above the packed erythrocytes following centrifugation; consists primarily of leukocytes and thrombocytes _____

24. Lepto cytes with a peripheral ring of cytoplasm surrounded by a clear area and a dense central rounded area of pigment _____

25. Leukocyte of avian, reptile, and some fish species containing prominent eosinophilic granules; functionally equivalent to the mammalian neutrophil _____

26. Neoplastic cells in the blood or bone marrow _____

27. Platelet; cytoplasmic fragment of bone marrow megakaryocyte _____

28. Presence of fatty material in plasma or serum _____

29. Procedure for classifying cells to determine relative percentages of each cell type present in a peripheral blood or bone marrow sample _____

30. Reddish appearance of cells or components of cells that have high affinity for stains with acid pH _____

31. Reduction in the oxygen-carrying capacity of blood due to a reduced number of circulating RBCs, reduced PCV, or a reduced concentration of hemoglobin _____

32. The closeness with which test results agree with the true quantitative value of the constituent _____

33. The magnitude of random errors and the reproducibility of measurements _____

34. Variable staining pattern; basophilia _____

35. White blood cell group that has no visible cytoplasmic granules _____

```
M H E O S I N O P H I L I A H E T E R O P H I L Q
H Y D I F F E R E N T I A L L P H A J N D G Q Z I
R P A V Q Z U A J O U Q L P M D J Z N B U F F Y Z
P O L Y C Y T H E M I A G L E U C O P E N I A A R
P C E B U P R M E G A K A R Y O C Y T E M M G C X
R H U G J A O K M T R C U G X D Q L T P M I R U R
E R K L S N P T H R O M B O C Y T O P E N I A N R
C O O A C C E H Y P E R S E G M E N T E D E N O E
I M C C H Y N T T J C L Y O D G L H T Z L A U R F
S I Y C I T I A U Q B X T U N D G Y J U I R L M R
I C T U S O A R V H G B K M K C C B O S A J O O A
O B O R T P P G J T E R K U Y O P R A I M J C C C
N S S A O E J E X R T B L W B T N M L Z L M Y H T
N W I C C N L T T I E C V M J B O I G N M H T R O
X O S Y Y I O C H J J T O U T R H J A K W A E O M
Z W R E T A W E D R P R I T H P N C M E N P V M E
I P L M E P Z L P B H N S C O M I V H B F J F I T
E C S O O Q V L L T V W Y R U D F L E E U S Y C E
A L T Q R C Z S O J J L T N X L Z M M G P X C D R
K F I E J A Y B Z G O U O I U I O Z O R R W D G E
T I O P R O P T A P E N F G U T F C L R W Z D D F
A Z L N E U L G I N P O I K I L O C Y T O S I S P
U F Y J E M S N V C D U E B C C J E S T C B F O F
L E U K E M I A B A S O P H I L I A I P E S K U D
G F D W J O H A S P W W Y I H E M O S T A S I S M
```

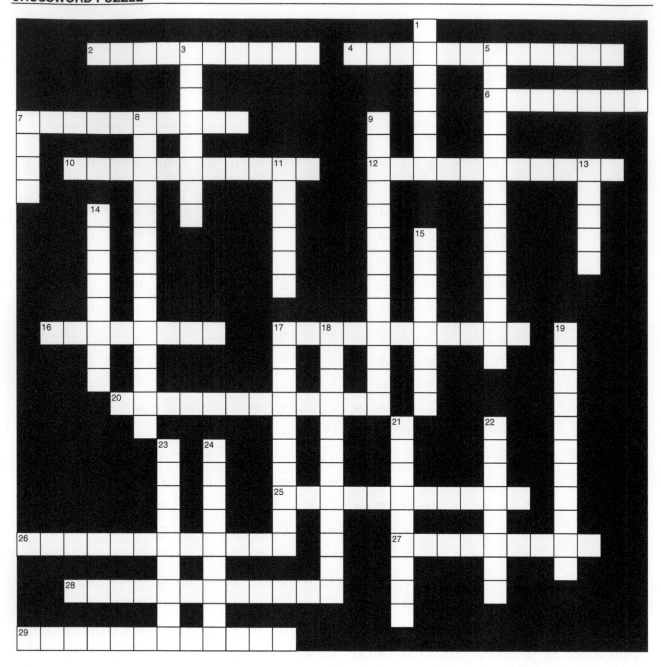

Across

2 An avian leukocyte functionally equivalent to a mammalian neutrophil. (10)

4 Having a high affinity for stains with an acid pH. (12)

6 Abnormal yellow discoloration of skin, mucous membranes, or plasma due to increased concentration of bile pigments. (7)

7 An increased number of basophils in peripheral blood. (10)

10 A blood sample that is obtained from an animal that has not eaten for a period of time is a ___ sample. (11)

12 A white blood cell with distinct cytoplasmic granules. (11)

16 The presence of neoplastic cells in blood or bone marrow. (8)

17 Erythrocytes that stain with less intensity because of a decreased hemoglobin concentration. (11)

20 An immature, anuclear, polychromatophilic erythrocyte stained with new methylene blue stain. (12)

25 A red blood cell fragment seen on a peripheral blood smear. (11)

26 DIC is a coagulation disorder that is characterized by depletion of ___ and coagulation factors. (12)

27 Destruction of erythrocytes. (9)

28 Decreased numbers of all blood cells and platelets in a peripheral blood sample. (12)

29 The ___ cell count is the procedure used to classify cells to determine the relative percentage of each white blood cell type present on a peripheral blood smear. (12)

Down

1 The presence of fatty material in plasma or serum. (7)

3 The arrangement of erythrocytes in stacks or columns as seen on a peripheral blood smear. (8)

5 The presence of abnormal cell shapes. (14)

7 A ___ cell is an immature granulocyte with a nucleus that has parallel sides with no nuclear lobes or indentation. (4)

8 Describes a neutrophil with more than five nuclear lobes. (14)

9 The large bone marrow cell from which thrombocytes are formed. (13)

11 A reduction in the oxygen-carrying capacity of blood. (6)

13 Döhle bodies are seen in ___ neutrophils. (5)

14 The ___ value is the number of each type of leukocyte in peripheral blood calculated using the relative percentage and total white blood cell count. (8)

15 The closeness with which test results agree with the true quantitative value of the constituent. (8)

17 Stopping the flow of blood through coagulation. (10)

18 An increase in the number of circulating erythrocytes. (12)

19 An abnormal decrease in neutrophils in peripheral blood. (11)

21 The presence of increased numbers of immature neutrophils in a peripheral blood sample. (2 words) (9)

22 A thrombocyte is a/an ___. (8)

23 A target cell is also called a/an ___. (9)

24 The layer of leukocytes and thrombocytes that lies on top of the packed erythrocytes in a spun hematocrit tube. (2 words) (9)

8 Clinical Chemistry and Serology

LEARNING OBJECTIVES

After reviewing this chapter, the reader will be able to:
- Describe methods used to collect samples of blood for laboratory examination
- Discuss ways in which diagnostic samples are prepared for laboratory examination
- Differentiate between serum and plasma
- List and describe equipment needed for clinical chemistry and serology testing
- State the advantages, disadvantages, and limitations of various models of clinical chemistry analyzers
- Describe the principles of operation of various chemistry and electrolyte analyzers
- List and describe the indications for and types of tests used in clinical chemistry testing
- List and describe the biochemical assays commonly performed to assess liver, kidney, and pancreatic function
- List the major intracellular and extracellular electrolytes and describe their roles in mammalian physiology
- Describe the roles of the white blood cells in the immune system
- List the types of immunologic tests and describe the test principles employed by those tests
- Discuss methods used to verify accuracy of laboratory test results

DEFINITION

Define the following terms:

1. Antigen

_____

_____

2. Azotemia

_____

_____

3. Cholestasis

_____

_____

4. Control

_____

_____

5. Cytokines

_____

_____

6. Electrolyte

_____

_____

7. Humoral immunity

_____

_____

8. Immunoglobulin

_____

_____

9. Standard

_____

_____

10. Titer

_____

_____

MATCHING

Match the following.

_____ 1. Coating of helminth parasites for destruction by eosinophils

_____ 2. Neutralization of microbes and toxins

_____ 3. Fetal and neonatal immunity by passive transfer across placenta and in colostrum

_____ 4. Protection of respiratory, intestinal, and urogenital tracts

_____ 5. Mucosal immunity

_____ 6. Activation of complement

_____ 7. Immediate hypersensitivity reactions, such as allergies and anaphylactic shock

A. IgG

B. IgM

C. IgE

D. IgA

E. IgD

SHORT ANSWER

1. List at least six tests of liver function.

    1. _____
    2. _____
    3. _____
    4. _____
    5. _____
    6. _____

2. List at least four tests used to evaluate the endocrine pancreas.

    1. _____
    2. _____
    3. _____
    4. _____

3. Differentiate between serum and plasma.

_____

_____

_____

4. Describe the general principle of photometry.

_____

_____

_____

_____

_____

5. Give the calculation used for a one-point calibration in a photometric analyzer.

_____

_____

_____

6. Describe the procedure for performing a total protein assay with a refractometer.

_____

_____

_____

_____

7. Describe the general principle of the ELISA reaction.

_____

_____

_____

_____

8. Differentiate between sensitivity, specificity, and predictive value.

_____

_____

_____

_____

9. List the electrolytes most commonly analyzed in samples from veterinary patients.

_____

_____

_____

_____

_____

10. Name two immunologic tests that are based on the principles of cell-mediated immunity.

_____

_____

_____

TRUE OR FALSE

1. _____ Glucose levels are increased in preprandial samples.

2. _____ Samples that are hemolyzed, icteric, or lipemic may yield inaccurate results with many of the automated analyzers.

3. _____ Endpoint assays are used for enzyme assays or when the reagent is enzyme based.

4. _____ Liver function tests referred to as the "leakage enzyme tests" include AST, ALT, and ALP.

5. _____ Total serum protein concentrations include all plasma proteins except fibrinogen and certain other coagulation proteins.

6. _____ Dehydrated animals usually have elevated total protein values.

7. _____ Severe hepatic insufficiency leads to increased albumin levels.

8. _____ Unconjugated bilirubin is also referred to as indirect bilirubin.

9. _____ Cholestasis causes backup of bile acids into blood.

10. _____ Cholesterol levels are frequently elevated in animals with hypothyroidism.

11. _____ AST assays are used primarily to evaluate the extent of skeletal muscle damage in the equine.

12. _____ In dogs, cats, and primates, the primary source of serum ALT is the hepatocyte.

13. _____ Dehydration can lead to azotemia.

14. _____ Uric acid is a the primary end product of nitrogen metabolism in mammals.

15. _____ Binding of glucose and serum proteins produces β-hydroxybutyrate.

FILL IN THE BLANK

1. Bile acids are produced from _____ in the liver.

2. Conjugated bilirubin is also referred to as _____ bilirubin.

3. Urobilinogen is broken down to _____ before being excreted in feces.

4. Globulins are a complex group of proteins that include all of the plasma proteins other than _____ and coagulation proteins.

5. Cholestatic tests include _____ and gamma glutamyl transferase (GGT).

6. In Dalmatian dogs, the liver is unable to convert _____ to allantoin.

7. Amylase is produced in a variety of tissues, including the _____, _____ _____, and _____.

8. The primary ketone produced in ketoacidosis is _____.

9. _____ is a serum enzyme that catalyzes the conversion of lactate to pyruvate.

10. _____ values are frequently used to monitor and develop prognostic indicators for critically ill patients.

11. _____ is the major cation of plasma and interstitial fluid.

12. _____ is the predominant extracellular anion and is an important component of serum osmolality.

13. The _____ system represents a series of enzymes that must react in a stepwise fashion in order to function.

14. The respiratory, digestive, and urinary systems contain groups of neutrophils, referred to as _____, which act as scavengers and function to phagocytize foreign substances.

15. _____ are often referred to as tissue macrophages and are capable of phagocytosis and antigen processing and presentation.

Identify the term described and then find the terms in the Word Search.

1. A biologic solution of known values used for verification of accuracy and precision of test results

   _____

2. A group of plasma proteins that function to enhance the activities of the immune system _____

3. A nonbiologic solution of an analyte, usually in distilled water, with a known concentration

   _____

4. A protein in the blood plasma that is essential for the coagulation of blood _____

5. Any condition in which bile excretion from the liver is blocked _____

6. Any substance that dissociates into ions when in solution _____

7. Compounds that are broken down to urobilin before being excreted in feces; may also be absorbed directly into the

   blood and excreted via the kidneys _____

8. Enzyme derived primarily from the pancreas that functions in the breakdown of starch _____

9. Enzyme-linked immunosorbent assay; an immunologic test _____

10. Icterus _____

11. Increased retention of urea in the blood _____

12. Insoluble pigment derived from the breakdown of hemoglobin, which is processed by hepatocytes

    _____

13. Molecule formed as a result of the irreversible reaction of glucose bound to protein _____

14. The principal end product of amino acid breakdown in mammals _____

15. Waste product formed during normal muscle cell metabolism _____

```
R  E  T  E  D  F  G  S  I  S  A  T  S  E  L  O  H  C
F  N  Y  U  N  G  F  U  Z  V  B  W  Q  C  F  Z  N  O
G  I  U  J  W  I  K  N  Q  G  G  E  W  I  G  H  M  N
B  M  M  N  O  H  N  R  M  R  A  Y  K  D  B  Y  F  T
M  A  B  L  E  Z  F  I  N  T  S  H  M  N  C  R  T  R
K  S  W  P  L  G  G  Q  T  Y  I  J  J  U  H  G  N  O
L  O  R  U  E  M  O  D  Y  A  L  K  N  A  P  D  E  L
J  T  G  J  C  A  C  N  H  P  E  P  Y  J  L  X  M  C
H  C  H  K  T  R  W  A  I  C  R  R  H  U  K  P  E  H
Y  U  K  R  R  G  K  D  G  R  F  H  C  P  I  L  L  E
T  R  T  G  O  I  U  R  T  B  B  N  H  O  N  K  P  M
P  F  H  V  L  Y  U  A  E  Y  Q  I  V  G  I  B  M  I
E  T  T  W  Y  H  I  D  Q  G  P  M  F  B  B  R  O  S
S  H  Y  F  T  M  Y  N  P  F  T  Y  P  J  U  R  C  T
A  G  P  Q  E  P  R  A  N  J  Y  E  G  T  R  F  G  P
L  N  Y  T  Q  O  N  T  Y  K  N  P  U  Y  I  T  J  A
Y  M  O  T  Y  K  A  S  E  L  E  D  Y  Q  L  G  H  E
M  Z  B  G  G  D  D  W  E  P  J  Q  T  Z  I  X  C  R
A  E  N  A  R  F  N  E  G  O  N  I  L  I  B  O  R  U
```

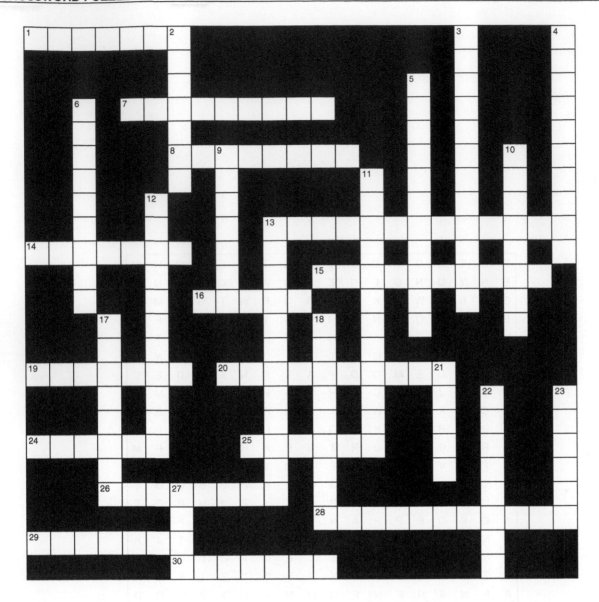

Across

1 The presence of fatty material in plasma or serum. (7)
7 The insoluble pigment derived from the breakdown of hemoglobin. It is processed by hepatocytes. (9)
8 A nonbiologic solution of an analyte, usually in distilled water, with a known concentration. (8)
13 Particles clumping together. (13)
14 A biologic solution of known values used for verification of accuracy and precision of test results. (7)
15 A small soluble protein that enhances the function of the immune system. (10)
16 A negatively charged ion. (5)
19 Immunity that involves production of specific antibodies is __ immunity. (7)
20 A group of plasma proteins that function to enhance the activities of the immune system. (10)
24 The __ test is an immunologic test designed to detect antibodies on the surface of erythrocytes or antibodies in plasma against erythrocytes. (6)
25 The pancreatic enzyme that functions in the breakdown of fats. (6)
26 The closeness with which test results agree with the true quantitative value of the constituent. (8)
28 Any substance that dissociates into ions when in solution. (11)
29 The immunity a newborn gets from drinking colostrum from its mother is __ immunity. (7)
30 Any substance capable of eliciting an immune response. (7)

Down

2 An enzyme produced primarily by the pancreas that functions in the breakdown of starch. (7)
3 Immune system mechanism involving actions of the cells of the immune system rather than antibodies. (2 words) (12)
4 A waste product formed during normal muscle cell metabolism. (10)
5 A small fat globule composed of protein and lipid. (11)
6 Soluble molecules that serve as mediators of cell responses. (9)
9 The group of plasma proteins that comprises the majority of protein in plasma. (7)
10 An immunoglobulin is also known as a/an __. (8)
11 The molecule formed as a result of the irreversible reaction of glucose bound to a protein. (12)
12 A condition where bile excretion from the liver is blocked. (11)
13 Any condition that results in the production of antibody against a body's own tissues. (12)
17 Increased retention of urea in blood. (8)
18 Immunologic __ is a state of being nonresponsive to antigens. (9)
21 The greatest dilution at which a patient sample no longer yields a positive result for the presence of a specific antibody. (5)
22 The complex group of plasma proteins that includes complement and transferrin. (8)
23 The type of immunity that results from an animal's production of antibody as a result of infection with an antigen or immunization. (6)
27 The principal end product of amino acid breakdown in mammals

Microbiology, Cytology, and Urinalysis

LEARNING OBJECTIVES

After reviewing this chapter, the reader will be able to:
- List and describe methods used to collect samples of body tissues and fluids for laboratory examination
- Describe methods used to prepare diagnostic samples for laboratory examination
- List and describe microbiologic tests commonly performed to identify bacterial, fungal, and viral pathogens
- Discuss procedures used in cytologic examination of body tissues and fluids
- List tests commonly performed in analyzing urine specimens
- Describe techniques of sample collection and processing for cytology and microbiology samples
- Identify common normal cells in cytology samples
- Identify common abnormal cells in cytology samples
- Describe methods for differentiation of inflammatory and neoplastic cytology samples

SHORT ANSWER

1. List three methods of sample collection for microbiology.

    1. _____

    2. _____

    3. _____

2. Describe four components of a bacterial cell.

    1. _____

    2. _____

    3. _____

    4. _____

3. Define bacterial generation time.

    _____

    _____

    _____

4. What is the most common cause of diagnostic failure with microbiology samples?

    _____

    _____

5. How should samples from animals with suspected zoonoses be submitted?

    _____

    _____

6. What reagent should be used to prepare a solid tissue sample for fungal testing?

   _____

   _____

7. Name two types of dermatophyte test media.

   1. _____

   2. _____

8. Name the media broth that is commonly used for urine cultures.

   _____

9. The catalase test is used to help identify Gram _____ _____ and small Gram _____ _____.

   The reagent used for the catalase test is _____ _____.

10. Name three bacteria for which ELISA tests are available to help detect antibodies.

    1. _____

    2. _____

    3. _____

11. Name two methods of antimicrobial sensitivity testing.

    1. _____

    2. _____

12. The primary goal of cytology evaluation is differentiation of _____ and _____.

13. Which sample collection technique yields the most cells? Impression or scraping?

    _____

14. What type of collection technique is preferred for fistulated lesions?

    _____

15. Give one advantage and one disadvantage for using the "starfish smear" technique for cytology.

    Advantage _____

    Disadvantage _____

16. What is the preferred fixative for cytology specimens?

    _____

17. In a cytology sample neutrophils and macrophages should be evaluated for the presence of _____ or _____.

18. Malignant changes seen in neoplastic cells include:

_____

_____

_____

19. Exudates that contain intracellular bacteria are classified as _____.

20. List the five general categories of cytology samples.

    1. _____

    2. _____

    3. _____

    4. _____

    5. _____

21. What is the primary function of neutrophils?

_____

22. A typical mixed cell population would involve _____ and _____.

23. Neoplasia needs to be differentiated as either _____ or _____.

24. Malignant cells display at least _____ abnormal nuclear configurations.

25. Name two types of abnormal nuclear configurations that indicate malignancy.

    1. _____

    2. _____

26. List the three basic tumor categories seen in mammals.

    1. _____

    2. _____

    3. _____

27. Mesenchymal cell tumors are also referred to as _____.

28. Name the type of tumor that tends to be highly cellular and often exfoliates in clumps.

_____

29. Mast cells have prominent dark _____ granules, whereas melanoma cells have prominent dark _____ granules.

30. List four types of round cell tumors.

1. _____

2. _____

3. _____

4. _____

31. Define lymphadenitis.

_____

32. List three types of cells typically seen in vaginal cytology samples.

1. _____

2. _____

3. _____

33. List three methods used to collect semen for artificial insemination.

1. _____

2. _____

3. _____

34. List two sperm head abnormalities and two sperm tail abnormalities that may be observed.

1. _____

2. _____

3. _____

4. _____

35. Why is it crucial that histology fixatives work rapidly and penetrate tissues?

_____

_____

_____

36. List four commonly used histology fixatives.

   1. _____

   2. _____

   3. _____

   4. _____

37. List three clearing agents that can be used for histology samples.

   1. _____

   2. _____

   3. _____

38. Describe the paraffin preparation of a histology sample.

   _____

   _____

   _____

39. List the components of the urinary system.

   _____

   _____

   _____

40. List the components of a kidney's nephron.

   _____

   _____

   _____

41. Define renal threshold.

   _____

   _____

42. List four methods of urine collection.

   1. _____

   2. _____

   3. _____

   4. _____

43. Two urine collection methods suitable for urine cultures are _____ and _____.

44. Why should manual expression of an obstructed bladder be avoided?

_____

_____

45. List six changes to urine as it sits at room temperature for more than 1 hour.

1. _____

2. _____

3. _____

4. _____

5. _____

6. _____

46. Gross examination of urine should include evaluation of color, _____, _____, and

_____.

47. Normal urine output for both canines and felines is _____ cc/pound in 24 hours.

48. Which urine dipstick tests may be unreliable for some veterinary species?

_____

49. Physiologic (nonpathogenic) proteinuria can occur with _____ or _____ _____

due to increased permeability of the _____ to plasma proteins.

50. Glucose in the urine is called _____ or _____.

51. List six causes of ketonuria.

1. _____

2. _____

3. _____

4. _____

5. _____

6. _____

52. Define hematuria.

_____

_____

53. Define hemoglobinuria.

_____

_____

54. How can hemoglobinuria be differentiated from hematuria?

_____

_____

55. Squamous epithelial cells originate in the _____ _____, _____, vagina, or

_____.

56. Myoglobinuria is usually seen in horses with _____.

57. In concentrated urine, erythrocytes will _____.

58. Define "ghost cells."

_____

_____

59. Where do transitional epithelial cells originate?

_____

_____

60. An increase in the number of _____ epithelial cells in the urine suggests inflammation.

61. Where do urinary casts originate?

_____

_____

62. How are granular casts formed?

_____

_____

63. The _____ and _____ of the urine affect the formation of crystals.

64. Name the type of urine crystal often referred to as triple phosphate.

_____

65. Calcium carbonate crystals are normal findings in the urine of _____ and _____.

66. Describe the shape of calcium carbonate crystals.

_____

_____

67. Name the type of urinary crystal most commonly associated with ethylene glycol poisoning.

_____

68. What breed of dog often has a metabolic defect that causes urinary uric acid crystal formation?

_____

69. Name and describe the urinary crystal often seen in animals with portosystemic shunts.

_____

_____

_____

70. Bacteria in urine should be reported as _____, _____, or _____.

TRUE OR FALSE

If false, change the statement to make it true.

1. _____ Aseptic technique is critical when collecting microbiology samples.

2. _____ Fungal mycelia grow into matted structures known as hyphae.

3. _____ Formalin fumes can render samples unsatisfactory for analysis.

4. _____ Carbon dioxide released by dry ice may kill bacteria and viruses.

5. _____ All bacteria that contain capsules are pathogenic.

6. _____ Most pathogenic bacteria should be incubated at room temperature (25° C).

7. _____ Triple-sugar-iron media requires Kovac's reagent.

8. _____ Microbiology samples collected after medical treatment starts produce better results.

9. _____ Some cytology samples require centrifugation in order to concentrate cells.

10. _____ Inflammatory specimens contain primarily tissue cells while neoplastic specimens contain primarily neutrophils and macrophages.

11. _____ For impression smears from active lesions, an initial impression should not be made until after cleaning the lesion.

12. _____ All fine needle aspirate sites should be surgically prepped before sample collection.

13. _____ Soft tissue masses require large-bore needles for aspiration.

14. _____ A line smear sample should have a feathered edge similar to blood smears.

15. _____ Longer fixative times improve staining quality and do not harm cytology samples.

16. _____ Cytology samples should be scanned on low magnification to ensure stain quality.

17. _____ Inflammatory exudates have low total protein values due to their high cellular content.

18. _____ It is usually not necessary to collect samples from hemorrhagic lesions.

19. _____ Neoplasia is indicated when cells present are of the same tissue origin.

20. _____ Benign neoplasia is represented by hyperplasia, but cells are of the same type and are relatively uniform in appearance.

21. _____ Inflammation always indicates malignancy.

22. _____ Normal lymph nodes usually have relatively even percentages of small, intermediate, and large lymphocytes.

23. _____ Optimal mating times can be determined based exclusively on vaginal cytology.

24. _____ Semen must be protected from temperature changes, water, and disinfectants.

25. _____ Live sperm stain pink/red with eosin stain.

26. _____ Most histology fixatives are capable of penetrating 2 to 4 mm per 24 hours.

27. _____ The ureter leaves the kidney at the renal pelvis.

28. _____ Each loop of Henle is surrounded by a Bowman capsule.

29. _____ Collecting tubules of the nephron drain urine into the renal pelvis to the opening of the ureter.

30. _____ The most concentrated urine sample is one collected after exercise.

31. _____ Urine from an intact bitch in proestrus may contain red blood cells.

32. _____ If refrigerated, urine samples should be warmed to body temperature before analysis.

33. _____ Alteration in the concentrating ability of the kidneys is an early indicator of renal tubular damage.

34. _____ Urine dipstick analysis should be performed on well-mixed, room temperature, and chemically preserved urine.

35. _____ Protein is normally present in very low quantities in urine.

36. _____ Nursing herbivores have acidic urine from the consumption of milk.

37. _____ Bilirubinuria is normal in all species except canines.

38. _____ Hemolytic diseases can cause bilirubinuria.

39. _____ A positive occult blood reading is most commonly associated with hemoglobinuria.

40. _____ Up to 5 RBC/HPF and 5 WBC/HPF is considered normal in urine.

41. _____ Squamous epithelial cells are common findings in cystocentesis urine samples.

42. _____ Casts dissolve in acidic urine.

43. _____ Urinary casts are formed due to slow-moving filtrate through the renal tubules.

44. _____ The presence of granular casts usually indicates severe kidney damage.

45. _____ Amorphous urate crystals appear as granular precipitate in alkaline urine.

46. _____ Urine obtained by cystocentesis is often contaminated by bacteria.

47. _____ Abdominocentesis does not require surgical prep. Thoracentesis does require surgical prep.

48. _____ Gamma hemolysis indicates partial destruction of red blood cells.

49. _____ Alpha hemolysis appears as a greenish haze.

50. _____ Beta hemolysis indicates no destruction of red blood cells.

MATCHING

Match the following.

1. _____ Pyknosis

2. _____ Epithelial cell tumor

3. _____ Cocci

4. _____ Karyhorrexis

5. _____ Bacillus

6. _____ Mesenchymal cell tumor

7. _____ Fungi

8. _____ Round cell tumor

9. _____ Bacteria

10. _____ Karyolysis

A. Round bacteria
B. Histiocytoma
C. Prokaryotic
D. Condensed nucleus
E. Eukaryotic
F. Carcinoma
G. Rod-shaped bacteria
H. Sarcoma
I. Fragmented nucleus
J. Lysed nucleus

Match the description of semen with the evaluation appropriate to the description.

1. _____ Distinct vigorous swirling

2. _____ Barely discernible swirling

3. _____ Moderate slow swirling

4. _____ Lack of obvious swirling

A. Fair
B. Good
C. Poor
D. Very Good

Match the term on the left to the definition on the right.

1. _____ Alpha hemolysis
2. _____ Pollakiuria
3. _____ Anuria
4. _____ Benign
5. _____ Polyuria
6. _____ Beta hemolysis
7. _____ Carcinoma
8. _____ Karyorrhexis
9. _____ Effusion
10. _____ Purulent
11. _____ Granulomatous
12. _____ Hyperplasia
13. _____ Sarcoma
14. _____ Isosthenuria
15. _____ Transudate
16. _____ Metastasis
17. _____ Neoplasia
18. _____ Suppurative
19. _____ Oliguria
20. _____ Urolithiasis

A. Complete destruction of red blood cells
B. Tumors of epithelial cell origin
C. Purulent
D. Calculi (stones) in the urinary tract
E. Urine specific gravity equal to glomerular filtrate
F. Neoplastic cells in areas other than originating tissue
G. Effusion with low TP and low TNCC
H. Decreased urine volume
I. Increased urine volume
J. Partial destruction of red blood cells
K. Nonmalignant tumor or growth
L. Fragmentation of a cell nucleus
M. Absence of urine
N. Containing, discharging, or producing pus
O. Generic term to describe any growth or tumor
P. Increase in frequency of urination
Q. Cancer arising from cells of connective tissue
R. Increase in the number of cells of an organ or tissue
S. Excess fluid in a tissue or body cavity
T. Inflammatory condition characterized by high numbers of macrophages

COMPLETE THE CHART

Fill in the blanks on the charts below.

Fluid	Inflammatory	TNCC	Total Protein
Transudate		<500/µl	
Modified transudate	No		2.5-5.0 g/dl
	Yes	>3000/µl	>3.0 g/dl

Type of Culture Media	Description	Example
Selective		MacConkey EMB
	Contains specific growth factors for bacteria with strict nutrient requirements	
Differential		

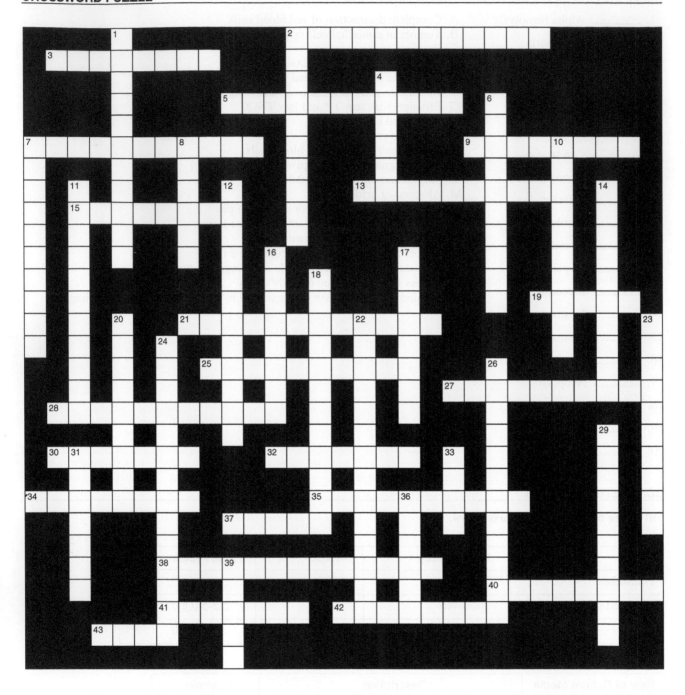

Across

2 Organisms that have optimal growth at elevated temperatures. (12)

3 Containing pus. (8)

5 An organism requiring high levels of carbon dioxide for growth. (11)

7 An increase in the number of cells of an organ or tissue. (11)

9 A staining procedure for demonstrating presence of microorganisms that are not readily decolorized by acid after staining; a characteristic of certain bacteria, particularly *Mycobacterium* and *Nocardia*. (2 words) (8)

13 Lymphadenitis is an inflammation of one or more __ __. (2 words) (10)

15 Decreased amount of urine being produced. (8)

19 Round-shaped bacteria. (5)

21 A group of cutaneous mycotic organisms commonly known as ringworm fungi. (12)

25 The presence of neoplastic cell in areas of the body other than where they originated. (10)

27 Fastidious pathogens require __ culture media to meet their growth requirements. (10)

28 A __ anaerobe does not require oxygen for survival but can survive in the presence of oxygen. (11)

30 Rod-shaped bacteria. (7)

32 A protein-rich, cellular fluid accumulation resulting from an inflammatory process. (7)

34 Exfoliative cytology that studies cells shed from body __. (8)

35 The area of no bacterial growth around an antimicrobial disk is called the zone of __. (10)

37 The type of hemolysis characterized by partial destruction of blood cells on a blood agar; evident as a greenish zone around the bacterial colony. (5)

38 Variation in the size of the nuclei in cells of a sample. (13)

40 Excessive fluid in a tissue or body cavity. (8)

41 __ bacteria inhabit the intestinal tract. (7)

42 Condensed nuclear chromatin in a degenerating cell. (8)

43 A seaweed extract used to solidify culture media. (4)

Down

1 Another word for purulent. (11)

2 An effusion characterized by low protein concentration and low total nucleated cell counts. (10)

4 Removal of cells or tissues for microscopic or chemical examination. (6)

6 A phagocytic cell derived from a monocyte. (10)

7 Hemoglobinuria describes the presence of free __ in urine. (10)

8 Absence of urine. (6)

10 Bacteria with complex growth or nutritional requirements are said to be a/an __ organism. (10)

11 Abnormally frequent urination. (11)

12 Fragmentation of a cell nucleus. (12)

14 The __ index is a measure of the degree of light bending as it passes from one media to another, relative to air. (10)

16 An enzyme that initiates the chemical reaction that breaks down hydrogen peroxide into water and oxygen. (8)

17 The act of puncturing a body cavity or organ with a hollow needle to draw out fluid. (8)

18 A condition where the urine specific gravity approaches that of the glomerular filtrate. (12)

20 Abnormally large volume of urine being produced. (9)

22 The microscopic study of diseased tissues. (14)

23 Carcinomas are tumors of __ cell origin. (10)

24 Specific gravity is the weight of a quantity of liquid compared with that of an equal amount of __ __. (2 words) (14)

26 Hematuria describes the presence of intact __ in urine. (12)

29 A sarcoma is a cancer that arises from __ tissues. (10)

31 In the presence of oxygen. (7)

33 The type of hemolysis characterized by complete destruction of red blood cells on a blood agar that creates a clear zone around the bacterial colony. (4)

36 A tumor that is not malignant is said to be __. (6)

39 Blood agar is usually made with __ blood. (5)

10 Veterinary Parasitology

LEARNING OBJECTIVES

After reviewing this chapter, the reader will be able to:
- List common internal parasites of domestic animals
- List common external parasites of domestic animals
- Discuss life cycles of common parasites of domestic animals
- Describe treatment and control strategies for common parasites of domestic animals
- Describe procedures used to diagnose parasites

TRUE OR FALSE

1. _____ The organism that the parasite lives in or on is called its host.

2. _____ All protozoa are parasitic.

3. _____ Trematodes lack a body cavity.

4. _____ Nematodes are commonly called roundworms because of their cylindrical body shape.

5. _____ The thorax of insects may have one or two pair of functional wings.

6. _____ Fleas demonstrate incomplete metamorphosis.

7. _____ Some adult flies glue their eggs to the hairs of the host.

8. _____ Ticks are arachnids.

9. _____ Most mite infestations are transmitted by indirect contact with an infested animal.

10. _____ Mites can be divided into two groups.

11. _____ Yellowish discoloration of feces can signify infection.

12. _____ Fecal direct smears are the most complicated of the evaluation process.

13. _____ Centrifugal flotation is more sensitive than simple flotation.

14. _____ The modified Knott's technique is a rapid method of microfilariae detection.

15. _____ Mite infestations are usually initially generalized.

FILL IN THE BLANK

1. Normal stool should be _____ yet _____.

2. Trematodes pass through several different _____ _____.

3. Most parasitic eggs have a specific gravity between _____ and _____ g/ml.

4. Some parasites produce _____ _____.

5. When herd studies are conducted, individual samples are taken from at least _____.

6. Buffy coat smear is a concentration technique for detection of _____ and _____ in white blood cells.

7. Direct drop is the least accurate heartworm test due to _____.

8. ELISA tests are highly accurate and precise and can detect _____ _____.

9. *Tritrichomonas foetus* is a _____ protozoan.

10. Fleas are laterally compressed _____ insects.

11. Flea larvae feed on _____ _____.

12. Organisms in the phylum Arthropoda are characterized by the presence of _____ _____.

13. Parasites residing on the surface of the host are called _____.

14. Trematodes are unsegmented and _____.

15. Cestode eggs contain a fully developed _____.

MATCHING

Match the following 20 terms to the description below.

_____ 1. Trematodes

_____ 2. Flagella

_____ 3. Undulatory ridges

_____ 4. Ectoparasite

_____ 5. Endoparasite

_____ 6. Commensalism

_____ 7. Mutualism

_____ 8. Parasitism

_____ 9. Cestodes

_____ 10. Scolex

_____ 11. Proglottids

_____ 12. Strobila

_____ 13. Gravid

_____ 14. Scutum

_____ 15. Demodex

_____ 16. Sarcoptic mange

_____ 17. *Cheyletiella*

_____ 18. *Otodectes*

_____ 19. *Oxyuris*

_____ 20. Microfilaria

A. Segments
B. Contains eggs
C. Loss of hair and intense pruritus
D. Pinworms
E. Heartworm larvae
F. Body
G. Whiplike structure
H. Organism that lives on another organism
I. Both organisms benefit
J. Head of a cestode
K. Organism that lives in another organism
L. One organism benefits; the other is harmed
M. Small snakelike waves that form in the cell membrane
N. Flatworms that lack a body cavity
O. Mite living in the external ear canal of dogs and cats
P. Walking dandruff
Q. Burrowing mite that lives in the hair follicles and sebaceous glands of the skin
R. Hard chitinous covering
S. Multicellular organisms that lack a body cavity
T. One organism benefits; other is unaffected

SHORT ANSWER

1. The three regions of the tapeworm are _____, _____, and _____.

2. The life cycle of nematodes follows a standard pattern of developmental stages; name them _____, _____, _____.

3. Diagnostic stages of nematodes are typically found in these four places _____, _____, _____, _____.

4. The three phyla in the kingdom animalia that have veterinary significance _____, _____, _____.

5. Name four organelles for locomotion _____, _____, _____, _____.

6. Phylum Sarcodina includes _____ and _____.

7. Explain direct life cycle.

_____

_____

8. Explain indirect life cycle.

_____

_____

9. Name three distinct body regions of an insect _____, _____, _____.

10. Arachnids include _____, _____, _____, and _____.

11. Name four problems caused by biting flies _____, _____, _____, _____.

12. Name the two main classifications of ticks _____, _____.

13. Name the two main classifications of mites _____, _____.

14. Describe the method used to recover ova of *Oxyuris* (pinworms).

_____

_____

_____

_____

15. Name materials needed for a direct smear _____, _____, _____, _____.

MULTIPLE CHOICE

1. A fecal smear should be:
   a. thick
   b. thin
   c. watery
   d. dry

2. To prepare a fecal smear for centrifugation you should use
   a. 3 to 6 g of feces
   b. 2 to 5 g of feces
   c. quarter size amount
   d. half dollar size amount

3. Materials for fecal culture include:
   a. glass jar
   b. charcoal
   c. wooden tongue depressor
   d. all of the above

4. Diagnostic trematodes have a simple digestive tract. Which two components are included in that digestive tract?
   a. mouth
   b. esophagus
   c. intestine
   d. stomach

5. Two groups in Phylum Platyhelminths that are important to veterinarians are:
   a. cestodes
   b. *Babesia*
   c. trematodes
   d. a and b
   e. a and c

6. A vector can be:
   a. mechanical
   b. biologic
   c. environmental
   d. a and b

7. Cestodes lack a digestive tract. Nutrients are absorbed through:
   a. blood
   b. body wall
   c. kidney
   d. liver

8. A cestode intermediate host could be:
   a. trout
   b. robin
   c. owl
   d. bee

9. Thorny head worms are found in which two of these animals?
   a. cats and dogs
   b. pigs and dogs
   c. birds and fish
   d. horses and goats

10. Arachnids have how many pairs of legs and how many body regions?
    a. 4, 1
    b. 8, 2
    c. 4, 2
    d. 4, 3

Unscramble each of the clue words.
Copy the letters in the numbered cells to other cells with the same number.

DORHAPORT

1

DADREOMLWRB

3

DECTOSE

TOERICSEAPAT

2

ATOASIDREPNE

4

FOLIRPIMCAIA

6

SOYCOT

CEOSXL

TADREOMET

7

SOTYRPOCS

5

1	2	3	4	5		U		U	
1	2	3	4	5		6		7	

Identify the term described and then find the terms in the Word Search.

1. Life cycle stage of trematodes that develops in the intermediate host _____

2. Organism in the order Cestoda; tapeworms _____

3. Parasitic larvae of mites _____

4. An insect of the taxonomic order Diptera (flies); most adults contain a single pair of wings _____

5. Dormant form of a bacterium _____

6. Blood-sucking parasites of dogs, cats, rodents, birds, and people _____

7. Any of several procedures for concentrating helminth eggs by use of a liquid of sufficiently high specific gravity _____

8. Trematode _____

9. Parasitic roundworm (*Dirofilaria immitis*) _____

10. Chewing or sucking parasitic insects _____

11. Life cycle stage of a protozoal parasite that results from asexual reproduction _____

12. Infestation with larvae (maggots) of dipterans _____

13. Roundworm _____

14. The egg stage of lice bound to hair or feather shaft of the host _____

15. Fluke species _____

16. Any of a large group of one-celled organisms; *Giardia* and *Toxoplasma* are examples _____

17. Description of mange that is caused by a tiny burrowing mite called *Sarcoptes scabiei* _____

18. Opposite of flotation; what is left when the supernatant is poured off. _____

19. Organism in the phylum Trematoda; commonly referred to as a fluke _____

20. Any organism that transmits a disease-causing organism to new hosts _____

```
F E F C B V S J I I N M N B V V X M T S
P O N Z H A A I A V V A Z Z S N Y M A U
Y Y X D E I S E J N N T R S Y I K K D M
R C G L O E G C Q J I U S E A N V M T I
L O F D H S H G F Z V T E S T S U B K N
S A T R V W P M E X I D I A N P Q W J O
P O K C J Q Q O E R O S L U C E I U U G
R H J T E N H D R T S Y Q H Y K B D A A
O E W D J Y O B A E S M N Q X D L O I R
T K N J N T B M V A F C M S J H E V R A
O U Q Z A V E C R S M N W B R N F C A P
Z L O M B R I C T I K B I X O H F H C G
O F E F T P O N P K M R A U N E A S R O
A N V Q R P M E R O Z O I T E A Q C E R
J N O I T A T O L E H C C A V R J P C R
S G O I C S Y S G M A P S I E T K S E D
H Z C X W R H U A X T J S A B W H H E D
V T T U E D B A A J E T W Y O O N V J K
S E D I M E N T W N J R M L M R S I F L
O C M H X K R E D O T S E C I M D Z N T
```

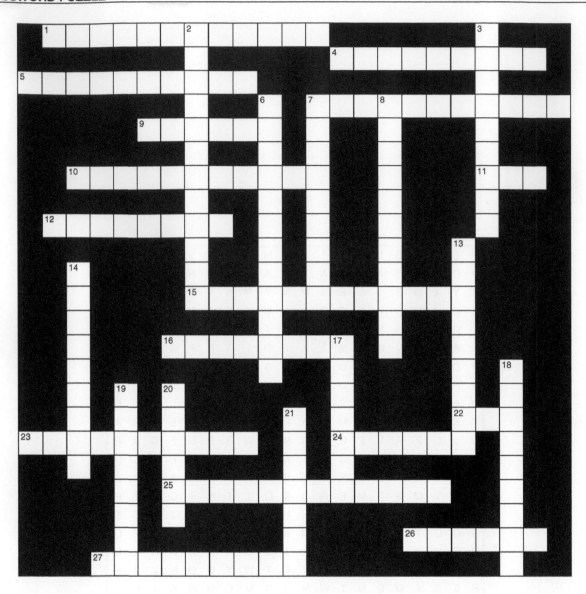

Across

1 Larval stage of the heartworm found in peripheral blood. (12)
4 Infective stage of some tapeworms. (9)
5 Tapeworm body segments. (10)
7 The motile form of a protozoan parasite. (11)
9 The common name for the larvae of some species of flies that are often found in cystlike subcutaneous sites with a fistula communicating to the outside environment. (6)
10 Fluid-filled larval stage of some cestodes. (11)
11 Most flies have __ pair(s) of wings as adults. (3)
12 Life cycle stage of a trematode that develops in the intermediate host. (8)
15 A parasite that resides on the surface of its host. (12)
16 A __ parasite lives part of its life cycle on its host and part off the host. (8)
22 The egg of a louse that is bound to the hair or feather shaft of the host. (3)
23 Tick paralysis is caused by introduction of a/an __ into the body by a female tick. (10)
24 Spore phase of some parasitic protozoa. (6)
25 A parasite that resides within a host's tissues. (12)
26 Any organism that transmits a disease-causing organism to a new host. (6)
27 Infestation with mites. (9)

Down

2 The __ host harbors the larval, immature, or asexual stages of a parasite. (12)
3 Dormant form of a bacterium. (9)
6 Parasites located in peripheral blood. (12)
7 The phylum to which flukes belong. (9)
8 Infestation with lice. (11)
13 The __ period is the time interval between infection with a parasite and demonstration of the infection. (9)
14 A lid or flap covering an opening commonly seen on trematode eggs. (9)
17 Tapeworms belong to the order __. (7)
18 The phylum to which ectoparasitic insects belong. (9)
19 A __ infection is one that can be spread from a nonhuman animal to a human. (8)
20 The head of a tapeworm. (6)
21 Infestation with maggots. (7)

Pharmacology and Pharmacy

After viewing this chapter, the reader will be able to:
- List the various categories of drugs and their clinical uses
- Identify dosage forms in which drugs are available
- Calculate drug dosages
- List and compare routes by which various types of drugs are administered
- Describe ways in which drugs exert their effect and affect body tissue
- Explain procedures used to safely store and handle drugs
- List the primary drugs affecting various body systems

FILL IN THE BLANK

1. Some drugs can be inactivated by violent shaking of the vial. An example of such a drug is _____.

2. Drug control records must include receipts for purchase or sale of controlled substances and must be maintained for _____ years.

3. For veterinarians to legally use, prescribe, or buy a controlled substance from an approved manufacturer or distributor, they must have obtained a _____ number from the DEA.

4. The ideal range of drug concentration minimizes detrimental effects and maximizes benefits. This is referred to as the _____ _____.

5. A drug's _____ is the amount of drug administered at one time.

6. The time between administrations of separate drug doses is referred to as the _____ _____.

7. Parenteral drugs are administered by _____.

8. Per os drugs are administered by _____.

9. A topically administered drug is administered by _____ it to the skin.

10. Accidental _____ injections can produce severe effects, such as seizures or respiratory arrest.

11. Intramuscular (IM) administration involves injecting the drug into a _____.

12. Subcutaneous (SC or SQ) injections are administered under the _____.

13. Intradermal (ID) injections are administered within the _____.

14. Intraperitoneal (IP) injections are administered into the _____.

15. Drugs or functions related to the stomach are called _____.

16. Drugs or functions related to the small intestines are referred to as _____.

17. Drugs and functions related to the colon are termed _____.

18. Activated charcoal adsorbs _____ to its surface, preventing them from contacting the bowel wall, thus allowing them to be passed out in the feces.

19. Anorexic cats often need an appetite stimulant. _____ is a serotonin antihistamine and _____ is a benzodiazepine that both work to stimulate appetite in cats but not in other species.

20. Lidocaine with _____ is designed for use as a local anesthetic, not as an antiarrhythmic drug.

21. A calcium channel blocker commonly used for hypertension in small animals is _____.

22. The drug of choice for maintaining long-term positive inotropic effects is _____.

23. Loop diuretics like _____ cause potassium to be excreted in the urine; prolonged use may result in hypokalemia.

24. The osmotic diuretic _____ is used to reduce cerebral edema associated with head trauma and as a diuretic for flushing absorbed toxins from the body.

25. The drug of choice for treating hypothyroidism is _____.

26. A common condition in cats that causes an increase in thyroid hormone production is called _____.

27. To treat hypoadrenocorticism two very similar sounding common glucocorticoid supplementations are used:

_____ and _____.

28. Livestock breeding systems use _____ to synchronize the estrous cycles of females, so that many animals can be artificially inseminated at the same time.

29. _____ _____ use increases the risk of cystic hyperplasia of the endometrium, endometritis, or pyometra.

30. To increase uterine contractions in animals with dystocia related to a weakened or fatigued uterus, the veterinarian commonly uses _____.

31. To produce short-term anesthesia, induce general anesthesia, control seizures, and euthanize animals, a _____ is often the drug of choice.

32. Drugs that kill or inhibit the growth of microorganisms or "microbes" such as bacteria, protozoa, viruses, or fungi are called _____.

33. The ability to survive in the presence of antimicrobial drugs is referred to as drug _____.

34. A residue is an accumulation of a drug, chemical, or its metabolites in animal tissues, which requires a _____ time be before the animal is slaughtered or the food products are to be marketed to people for food.

35. The "cillin" that is not be given per os because the gastric acid deactivates it is _____.

36. _____ are classified by generations, according to when they were first developed.

37. Topical antibiotic creams or ointments are often combined with polymyxin B, neomycin, and _____ to provide a broad spectrum of antibacterial activity.

38. Aminoglycosides are bactericidals effective against many aerobic bacteria; a common one used in veterinary clinics is _____.

39. _____ can cause arthopathies in immature, growing animals and should not be used in these animals.

40. An effective antibiotic against *Mycoplasma*, spirochetes such as *Chlamydia*, and rickettsia is _____.

41. Effective against many gram-positive aerobic cocci, _____ is approved only for use in dogs, cats, and ferrets.

42. *Giardia* (giardiasis) is a protozoa that causes intestinal disease, _____ is a commonly used treatment.

43. Because _____ is secreted into the renal tubule, it is a good choice for treating lower urinary tract infections.

44. Fungus that effects the skin, hair, nails, and claws is often treated with _____, which is a fungistatic.

45. Compounds that kill various types of internal parasites are called _____.

46. Collies and Collie cross-breeds should not receive _____ because it causes adverse reactions.

47. Amitraz was the first effective agent for treatment of _____ mange in dogs.

48. _____ interferes with development of the flea's chitin, which is essential for proper egg formation and development of the larval exoskeleton.

49. Drugs that relieve pain or discomfort by blocking or reducing the inflammatory process are called _____.

50. If the label of a vial specifies the active ingredient as dexamethasone, without mention of _____

_____, it is likely an alcohol solution.

51. In large doses or in sensitive animals, _____ can produce gastric ulcerations or decreased blood flow to the kidneys.

52. Aspirin has a half-life of _____ hours in people, approximately _____ hours in dogs, and _____ hours in cats.

53. Both dogs and cats are very sensitive to the OTC medications _____, _____, and _____, possibly developing liver and kidney failure and so are not generally recommended for clients to give to their pets.

54. Metabolites of _____ can have severe side effects; a single "extra-strength" tablet (500 mg) can kill an average-sized cat and cause hepatic necrosis in dogs.

55. _____ is the destruction of pathogenic microorganisms or their toxins.

56. Chemical agents that kill or prevent the growth of microorganisms on living tissues are called _____.

57. Chemical agents that kill or prevent the growth of microorganisms on inanimate objects are called _____.

58. The most common antiseptic applied to skin is _____ and usually is in a solution of _____%.

59. A common quaternary ammonium compound used to disinfect inanimate objects in the veterinary clinic is

_____ _____.

60. Two chemicals broadly effective as disinfectants used on skin are _____ and _____.

SHORT ANSWER

1. Describe the differences between a nonproprietary (generic) drug name and a proprietary (trademark) drug name.

_____

_____

2. Drug manufacturers and distributors are required to identify a controlled substance on its label with a capital C, followed by a Roman numeral, which denotes the drug's theoretical potential for abuse. Give the potential abuse and two examples of the drugs classified under each.

CI _____

_____

_____

CII _____

_____

CIII _____

_____

CIV _____

_____

CV _____

_____

Chapter 11 Pharmacology and Pharmacy

3. Pharmacokinetics involves absorption, distribution, metabolism, and elimination. Briefly explain what each of these entail and what organs, tissues, or vessels they interact with on their journey through the body.

Absorption

_____

_____

Distribution

_____

_____

Metabolism

_____

_____

Elimination

_____

_____

4. Emetics are drugs that induce vomiting. Answer the following questions about emetics:

A. Specifically why are they used?

_____

_____

B. What hazard is associated with their use?

_____

_____

C. Under what circumstances shouldn't they be used?

_____

_____

D. Which kind of drug works well as an emetic on a cat?

_____

_____

E. Which kind of drug works well as an emetic on a dog?

_____

_____

5. What disadvantages are associated with using narcotics as an antidiarrheal?

_____

_____

_____

_____

6. Answer the following questions about laxatives, lubricants, and stool softeners.

   A. What are the differences between irritant laxatives and bulk laxatives?

   _____

   _____

   B. How does mineral oil work on the colon?

   _____

   _____

   C. What does a stool softener do?

   _____

   _____

   D. How does lactulose work?

   _____

   _____

7. Which heart medication relaxes the blood vessels on the venous side of the circulation and may also help dilate coronary arterioles?

   _____

   _____

   _____

   _____

8. Describe the difference between a productive cough and a nonproductive cough.

   _____

   _____

   _____

   _____

9. Why is it important to tell clients not to use OTC cold medicines for the cat's cough?

   _____

   _____

   _____

   _____

10. What are the insulins of choice for maintaining diabetic dogs and cats?

    _____

    _____

11. Estradiol cypionate is used both on mares and small animals to:

    _____

    _____

Chapter 11 Pharmacology and Pharmacy

1. A 6-lb feline is prescribed amoxicillin at 5 mg/kg twice a day for 7 days. The oral medication has a concentration of 50 mg/ml. How many ml will the cat need per day?

2. A 30-lb Cocker Spaniel is to get a ketamine and diazepam induction IV with a dose of 0.025 ml/lb for each. How much ketamine and diazepam will you draw up?

3. A 1200-lb Holstein cow requires a ketoprofen injection. The veterinarian prescribes 1 mg/lb and the concentration is 100 mg/ml. How much ketoprofen will you give?

MATCHING

Drug formulations.

_____ 1. Solid dosage forms injected or inserted under the skin

_____ 2. Tablets and capsules

_____ 3. Drugs dissolve, release, and are absorbed by intestinal wall

_____ 4. Drug particles not dissolved in a liquid vehicle

_____ 5. Solutions of drugs with water and sugar

_____ 6. Administered via a needle and syringe

_____ 7. Alcohol solutions meant for topical application

_____ 8. Semisolid dosage forms that are applied to the skin

_____ 9. Drugs dissolved in sweetened alcohol

_____ 10. Drug dissolved in a liquid vehicle

_____ 11. Semisolid dosage forms given orally

A. Ointments
B. Elixirs
C. Suspension
D. Implants
E. Tinctures
F. Solution
G. Injectables
H. Solid
I. Pastes
J. Syrups
K. Suppositories

Antiemetics (match the drug name with the brand name).

_____ 1. Phenothiazine tranquilizers

_____ 2. Meclizine

_____ 3. Prochlorperazine

_____ 4. Metoclopramide

_____ 5. Chlorpromazine

_____ 6. Diphenhydramine

_____ 7. Dimenhydrinate

_____ 8. Cisapride

A. Compazine
B. Dramamine
C. PromAce
D. Propulsid
E. Reglan
F. Benadryl
G. Thorazine
H. Bonine

Match anesthetic drugs with their actions.

_____ 1. Cough control, GI-related, and colic pain

_____ 2. Long-term control of seizures and for euthanasia

_____ 3. Reversal of CNS depression from xylazine and dexmedetomidine

_____ 4. Inhalant anesthetic

_____ 5. Commonly used dissociative anesthetic

_____ 6. A strong narcotic analgesic often on a patch

_____ 7. CNS stimulant that increases respiration

_____ 8. Calming effect, decreased stimulus response, light analgesic

_____ 9. Benzodiazepine tranquilizer with good muscle relaxation

_____ 10. Laughing gas; weak analgesic

_____ 11. Phenothiazine tranquilizer; reduces anxiety

_____ 12. Potent, with long duration of analgesia

A. Ketamine
B. Barbiturates
C. Nitrous oxide
D. Isoflurane
E. Acepromazine
F. Fentanyl
G. Diazepam
H. Xylazine
I. Butorphanol
J. Buprenorphine
K. Doxapram
L. Yohimbine

WORD SEARCH

Identify the term described and then find the terms in the Word Search.

1. A drug dissolved in a liquid vehicle that does not settle out if left standing _____

2. A drug given intravenously as a single volume at one time _____

3. A drug in which the particles are suspended but not dissolved in the liquid vehicle _____

4. A drug that kills or inhibits the growth of microorganisms such as bacteria, protozoa, or fungi _____

5. A drug that paralyzes a worm but does not kill it _____

6. A drug that relieves pain or discomfort by blocking or reducing the inflammatory process _____

7. A reproductive hormone similar to progesterone _____

8. A solution of drug with water and sugar _____

9. A specific protein molecule on or in the cell that a drug will combine with _____

10. An alcohol solution meant for topical application _____

11. An altered drug molecule _____

12. An anthelminthic that kills the worm _____

13. An order from a licensed veterinarian directing a pharmacist to prepare a drug for use in a client's animal
_____

14. Another term for either antiseptics or disinfectants _____

15. Antimicrobial _____

16. Chemical agents that kill or prevent the growth of microorganisms on inanimate objects _____

17. Chemical agents that kill or prevent the growth of microorganisms on living tissue _____

18. Compounds that increase the fluidity of mucus in the respiratory tract by generating liquid secretions by respiratory tract cells _____

19. Directly neutralize acid molecules in the stomach or rumen _____

20. Drugs that increase urine formation and promote water loss _____

21. Drug that inhibits bronchoconstriction _____

22. Drug that reduces swelling of mucous membranes _____

23. Drugs or functions related to the colon _____

24. Drugs or functions related to the duodenum, jejunum, or ileum (small intestines) _____

25. Drugs or functions related to the stomach _____

26. Drugs that are used to control seizures _____

27. Drugs that induce vomiting _____

28. Drugs that reduce the perception of pain without loss of other sensations _____

29. Drugs used to stimulate an atonic rumen _____

30. General term used to describe compounds that kill various types of internal parasites _____

31. Given by injection _____

32. Glucocorticoid _____

33. Glucocorticoid _____

34. How a drug moves into, through, and out of the body _____

35. Inhibits bacterial replication _____

36. Inhibits protozoal replication _____

37. Kills bacteria _____

38. Kills fungi _____

39. Kills viruses _____

40. Movement of drug molecules from the site of administration into the systemic circulation _____

41. Opens (dilates) constricted vessels _____

42. Protein hormones secreted by gonadotrope cells of the pituitary gland, including FSH and LH _____

43. Size, frequency, and number of doses _____

44. Solution of drug dissolved in sweetened alcohol _____

45. Steroid hormones produced by the adrenal cortex of animals _____

46. The alteration of a drug by the body before eliminated _____

47. The period after drug administration during which the animal cannot be sent to market for slaughter and the eggs or milk must be discarded

48. Without a trademark or brand name; nonproprietary _____

124

```
C P M B Q L N B S T S C I T P E S I T N A T S Y E
I B R O B A S A A A N T I B I O T I C G B U D R M
R O W E P D N C X C T A R C G H E K M N S K I O I
E L N F S I M T N A T O T E I M Z S B P F M S T T
N U V S T C V E E G N E V S E R C I E E R T I A L
E S W I B U R R T C R V R T E I T N P U S S N M A
G L Z T L R N I H A S O I I S G S S M H C X F M W
G E I O S I B O P C B C T E C I N I A I W S E A A
R L O X D V D S I T S O G A O I N O T G M T C L R
N P U Q I I U T M T I L L N L A D E C F J N T F D
O W S C L R E A S Y A O K I T I N A B E N A A N H
I U C A O R N T C N Y M N O T I D L L X D R N I T
T B T I U C M I A I R V R D K E Y O U X C O T I I
P O O I G K O C A N T I C O N V U L S A N T S T W
R E D I C I M R E V C A C D F P M U B A M C C N P
O D O S A G E K T S V A T F S S R C Z L V E O A A
S D I C A T N A C I M E T S Y S N O N H U P L L R
B R E C E P T O R R C B R I I D S A G H R X O A E
A C I R E T N E A E E O M M N O O L R E T E N I N
U T A B X L I H V X H P I W I C Z O A T S H I C T
H Y B Z Z U P C K H G S T D I F T O I C O T C I E
A N T I M I C R O B I A L A S L U U T J G I I G R
D I O R E T S O C I T R O C B V Y G R O J I B N A
P G D I C I T N I M L W H T N A V D E E R X A U L
G O N A D O T R O P I N E N O S I T R O C P E F L
P U R Y S L A D I C I G N U F S O L U T I O N X Y
```

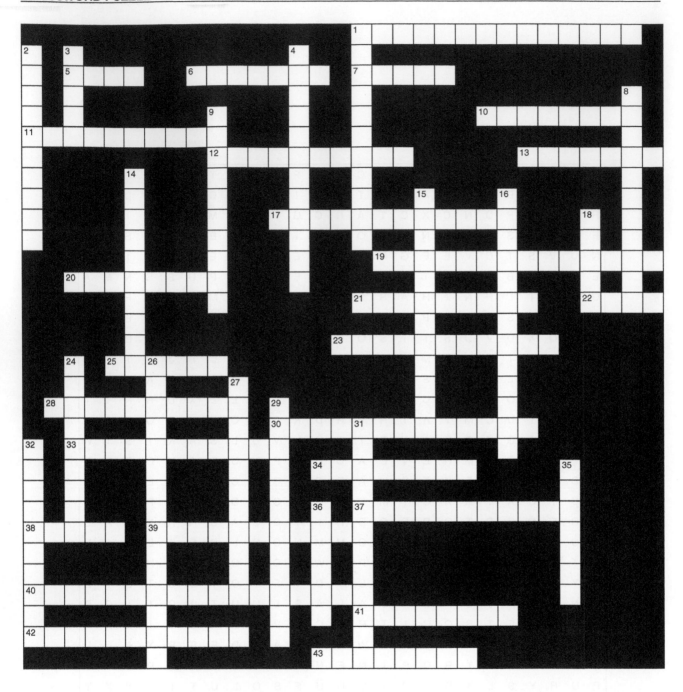

Across

1 A _____ level of a drug dose is below the ideal range of concentration and therefore does not produce the beneficial effect. (14)

5 Medications administered by mouth are _____ medications. (4)

6 A drug that is meant to be applied to the skin is a/an _____ drug. (7)

7 A semisolid dosage form given by mouth. (5)

10 A drug dissolved in a liquid vehicle that doesn't settle out if left standing. (8)

11 A drug in which there are particles suspended but not dissolved in a liquid vehicle. (10)

12 Movement of drug molecules from the site of administration into the systemic circulation. (10)

13 The _____ name of a drug is also called its nonproprietary name. (7)

17 The movement of a drug from the systemic circulation into tissues. (12)

19 Anything that inhibits bacterial replication. (14)

20 A drug that increases urine formation and promotes water loss. (8)

21 Positive _____ drugs increase the strength of contraction of the heart. (9)

22 The amount of a drug administered at one time. (4)

23 A drug used to stimulate an atonic rumen. (11)

25 A solution of a drug dissolved in sweetened alcohol. (6)

28 Any abnormal pattern of electrical activity in the heart. (10)

30 An injection made into a muscle mass. (13)

33 An injection made into a vein. (11)

34 The dosage _____ is the time between administrations of separate drug doses. (8)

37 A drug that increases the fluidity of mucus in the respiratory tract. (11)

38 A semisolid dosage form applied to the skin. (5)

39 An injection made within, not beneath, the skin. (11)

40 The alteration of a drug by the body before it is eliminated. (17)

41 An alcohol solution meant for topical application. (8)

42 Drug _____ is the removal of a drug from the body. (11)

43 The specific protein molecule on or in a cell with that a drug will combine. (8)

Down

1 A drug that is inserted into the rectum. (11)

2 A chemical agent that kills or prevents the growth of microorganisms on living tissue. (10)

3 A drug given intravenously as a single volume at one time. (5)

4 Anything that kills bacteria. (12)

8 Drugs that kill or inhibit the growth of microorganisms such as bacteria, protozoa or fungi. (11)

9 Drugs that reduce the perception of pain without loss of other sensations. (10)

14 The _____ time is the period after drug administration during which an animal cannot be sent to market for slaughter and the eggs or milk must be discarded. (10)

15 An injection made beneath the skin, but not into a muscle. (12)

16 A term synonymous with antibiotic. (13)

18 The acronym for a nonsteroidal antiinflammatory drug. (5)

24 A drug that paralyzes a worm but doesn't kill it. (9)

26 An injection made into the abdominal cavity. (15)

27 A drug that opens constricted vessels. (11)

29 A chemical agent that kills or prevents the growth of microorganisms on inanimate objects. (12)

31 General term used to describe compounds that kill various types of internal parasites. (12)

32 A drug that is administered using a syringe and needle is a/an _____ drug. (10)

35 Drugs that function in the small intestines are _____ drugs. (7)

36 A drug that induces vomiting. (6)

12 Pathology, Response to Disease, and Preventive Medicine

After reviewing this chapter, the reader will be able to:
- Describe ways in which tissues respond to injury
- List the phases of inflammation and the cells involved
- Describe ways in which injured tissues heal
- List and describe ways in which pathogens affect tissues
- Discuss types of immune responses
- Discuss the physiologic basis for vaccination
- Describe hypersensitivity reactions
- List and describe common zoonotic diseases and ways in which they can affect people
- Discuss methods used to control spread of zoonotic diseases
- Explain the general principles of epidemiology and their application to public health
- Explain the general principles of food hygiene and their application to public health
- Explain the general principles underlying disease prevention
- Discuss features of appropriate housing and nutrition for animals
- List and discuss types of vaccinations and schedules of vaccinations for domestic animal species
- Explain the principles of sanitation that relate to disease prevention
- Describe factors that predispose to disease
- Discuss general principles of incorporating a wellness program into a veterinary facility

SHORT ANSWER

1. The Shirmer Tear Test is used to identify what ocular condition? _____

2. Keratoconjunctivitis sicca and glaucoma can cause what symptom in pets? _____

3. A tonometer is used to screen patients for what disease? _____

4. Electrocardiographs and chest radiographs are used to evaluate a patient's _____.

5. *Giardia* and *Coccidia* are what type of parasites? _____

6. A differential blood film can be used to detect what three parasites? _____ _____

   _____

7. A profile is several tests put together. A coagulation profile includes a platelet count and what three other tests?

   _____ _____ _____

8. A CBC is an acronym for _____.

9. By what age should every patient have a baseline CBC chemistry panel drawn? _____

10. What three instruments are used during a physical examination? _____ _____

    _____

11. Wellness programs vary based on a patient's _____ and _____.

12. A complete physical examination should be performed how often? _____

13. Animals are predisposed to disease by what four means? _____ _____ _____ _____

14. The destruction of vegetative forms of bacteria on inanimate or nonliving objects is _____.

15. The destruction of all organisms, including bacteria and spores, is _____.

16. The prevention of infectious agent growth on living objects is _____.

17. Two examples of regularly administered preventive medications are? _____ _____

18. Veterinarians can offer to measure what type of titer before vaccinating a patient? _____

19. Vaccines that are recommended for all patients of a particular species are considered _____ vaccines.

20. Vaccines that are recommended based on a patient's lifestyle are considered a _____ vaccine.

21. Due to a growing concern for injection site sarcoma, it is recommended to vaccinate where on the patient's body? _____

22. CIRD is an acronym for what disease complex? _____

23. Canine influenza virus, canine parainfluenza virus, and *Bordetella bronchiseptica* are part of what disease complex? _____

24. Maternal antibodies to a disease can be transferred to the offspring through _____.

25. Rodents and rabbits are not routinely _____ because of a low risk for contracting disease.

26. A vaccine that consists of a weaker version of a pathogen is _____.

27. A vaccine that consists of whole killed or selected antigenic subunits is _____.

28. A vaccine that consists of a live, nonpathogenic virus into which the gene for a pathogen-related antigen has been inserted is _____.

29. Two forms of identification that cannot be removed are _____ and _____.

30. Diets improperly fed to the wrong species can cause _____ in animals.

31. Water containers develop _____, _____, or _____ when not sanitized regularly.

32. At what temperature are cleaned food and water dishes considered sanitized? _____

33. Food and water dishes should be sanitized how often? _____

34. Cages, pens, and stalls that are too small can lead to _____ behavior.

35. The rule of thumb for determining the adequate size for a pet enclosure is _____ times the body size.

36. One species can be a carrier of a disease that can be _____ to another.

37. To make a dilute bleach solution for sanitization, mix 1 part _____ to 20 parts _____.

38. Urine odors, ammonia levels, airborne bacteria, and viruses can be controlled with adequate _____.

39. Low humidity, air conditioning, and high air flow can cause _____ in animals.

40. Animals may become _____ or _____ if kept in direct sunlight.

41. All animals do better when there is a difference between _____ and _____ in their environment.

42. Ambient room temperature is between _____ and _____.

43. Preventive medicine prolongs the _____, improves the _____ of animals, and fosters a _____ relationship.

44. The goal of any preventive medicine program is to _____ incidence of disease.

45. Three major components of a preventive medicine program are _____, _____, and _____.

46. As part of preventive medicine, housing, diet, and environment are all considered _____.

47. As part of preventive medicine, cleanliness and disinfectants are considered _____.

48. Who is most susceptible to contracting a zoonotic disease? _____ _____

49. Veterinary professionals are at risk of contracting _____ diseases.

50. _____ can be implemented before a large outbreak of a zoonotic disease occurs.

51. _____ is a type of zoonosis that depends on an inanimate reservoir to maintain the cycle of infection.

52. An example of a saprozoonosis infection is _____, caused by *Toxocara* spp.

53. _____ is a type of zoonosis that is maintained by both invertebrate and vertebrate species.

54. An example of a metazoonosis infection is _____, which is spread by the mosquito.

55. _____ is a type of zoonosis that requires several cycles of disease, usually parasitic, to cause disease in several different vertebrates.

56. An example of a cyclozoonosis infection is _____, in which the hydatids become encysted.

57. A _____ is a living organism that transports an infectious agent.

58. _____ is the mode of transmission of an infectious agent from the reservoir to the host.

59. _____ transmission requires close association or contact between a reservoir of the disease and the susceptible host.

60. Disease can be spread via the _____ or _____ routes.

61. _____ are diseases that are transmitted between animals and people.

62. Who monitors foodstuff for the presence of residues and is responsible for inspection of food? _____

63. Who sets the limits for pesticide residues? _____

64. Who sets the limits for drug residues? _____

65. What does the acronym FDA stand for? _____

66. What does the acronym EPA stand for? _____

67. What does the acronym USDA stand for? _____

68. There are four types of allergic reactions. Which type occurs within minutes after exposure to the antigen? _____

Chapter 12 Pathology, Response to Disease, and Preventive Medicine

69. There are four types of allergic reactions. Which type is mediated by IgE antibodies on the surface of mast cells? _____

70. There are four types of allergic reactions. Which type involves the destruction of certain cells by neutrophils and macrophages? _____

71. There are four types of allergic reactions. Which type involves antigens and antibodies interacting to form immune complexes within various tissues? _____

72. There are four types of allergic reactions. Which type occurs hours after sensitized animals are again exposed to a particular antigen? _____

73. What type of immunity involves production of antibodies? _____

74. What type of immunity primarily involves actions of T lymphocytes? _____

75. Would skin and mucous membranes be considered a nonspecific or specific immune system defense mechanism? _____

76. Would antibodies and lymphocytes be considered a nonspecific or specific immune system defense mechanism? _____

77. The end result of tissue repair is _____ or _____.

78. What is the visible product of the inflammatory process? _____

79. Agents that cause an abnormal increase in the body temperature are called _____.

80. The study of disease is known as _____.

MATCHING

Match the following cells to their function.

_____ 1. Neutrophils

_____ 2. Eosinophils

_____ 3. Lymphocytes

_____ 4. Monocytes

A. Responsible for humoral antibody production
B. Primary function is phagocytosis
C. A more specific phagocytosis and lysosomal enzyme release
D. Become macrophages when they enter tissue at the site of inflammation

Match the following terms.

_____ 1. Wound

_____ 2. Parasites

_____ 3. Fibrosis tissue

_____ 4. Granulation tissue

_____ 5. Disease

_____ 6. Virus

A. Organisms that have adapted to live on or within a host organism
B. Any alteration from the normal state of health
C. An injury caused by physical means, with disruption of normal structures
D. Extremely small infectious agents that can cause disease in a wide variety of animals
E. A highly vascularized connective tissue that is only produced after extensive tissue damage
F. Primarily comprises dense fibrous connective tissue and collagen and contracts when mature

Match the cell type to its function.

_____ 1. B lymphocytes

_____ 2. T lymphocytes

A. Antibodies that are produced by plasma cells
B. Play a role in cell-mediated responses

Choose the vaccines for the species listed. Multiple selections are possible for each item.

1. Choose the canine vaccinations:
   a. Coronavirus
   b. *Chlamydia*
   c. Leptospirosis
   d. Strangles
   e. Brucellosis

2. Choose the canine vaccinations:
   a. *Porphyromonas*
   b. *Microsporum* spp.
   c. Leptospirosis
   d. Anthrax
   e. *Crotalus atrox*

3. Choose the feline vaccinations:
   a. Panleukopenia
   b. *Microsporum* spp.
   c. Leptospirosis
   d. Anthrax
   e. Rotavirus

4. Choose the feline vaccinations:
   a. Campylobacteriosis
   b. Rabies
   c. Adenovirus (CAV-1)
   d. Rhinotracheitis
   e. Rotavirus

5. Choose the equine vaccinations:
   a. Campylobacteriosis
   b. Rabies
   c. Adenovirus (CAV-1)
   d. Rhinotracheitis
   e. Rotavirus

6. Choose the equine vaccinations:
   a. Trichomoniasis
   b. Encephalomyelitis
   c. Brucellosis
   d. Rhinotracheitis
   e. Tetanus

7. Choose the goat vaccinations:
   a. Leptospirosis
   b. Encephalomyelitis
   c. Brucellosis
   d. Rhinotracheitis
   e. Tetanus

8. Choose the llama vaccinations:
   a. Trichomoniasis
   b. Leptospirosis
   c. Brucellosis
   d. Anthrax
   e. Tetanus

WORD SEARCH

Identify the term described and then find the terms in the Word Search.

1. Extremely small, nonliving infectious agent, ranging from 30 to 450 nm in diameter, that can cause disease in a wide variety of animals _____

2. The housing, diet, and environment of animals _____

3. An injury caused by physical means, with disruption of normal structures _____

4. Fever _____

5. White blood cells _____

6. Biologic products representing a pathogenic organism that stimulates immunity toward the pathogen

   _____

7. Environmental Protection Agency _____

8. Level of antibodies present in the serum (blood) _____

9. The usual food and drink consumed by an organism _____

10. A vaccine that consists of a live, nonpathogenic virus into which the gene for a pathogen-related antigen has been inserted _____

11. The act of inspecting something closely _____

12. The study of disease _____

13. Chemical substance that causes disease; produced in the cell walls of Gram-negative bacteria, they often stimulate the release of pyrogens by the host's cells _____

14. An inherent protective mechanism of the body; consists of nonspecific defenses and specific defenses

    _____

15. Ingestion of substances, including pathogens, by cells _____

16. Postmortem examination of an animal body _____

17. A relatively mild cutaneous hypersensitivity reaction such as hives _____

18. Visible product of the inflammatory process; usually composed of cellular debris, fluids, and cells that are deposited in tissues and on tissue surfaces _____

19. Living being that offers an environment for maintenance of the organism; not always necessary for the organism's survival _____

20. Capable of being transmitted from animals to human beings _____

21. The migration of certain nematodes through an organism's tissues and organs _____

```
V I R U S E P P Z O O I N E Q W E E R
I C B P S X A H U S B A N D R Y X T U
S O A H D A T A T I C M E P C V A C R
C M N A F M H G F D S I C A N B M O T
E J D G G H W O U N D G R T Z O O M I
R I N E T I C C C Y T R O H M L E Y C
A T I C H T Y Y R T R A P Y R E X I A
L E U K O C Y T E S I U S P E C U G R
L S Y S S R I O O T O P Y H C E D K I
A Z O O T I N S L O K L G A O R A I A
R L W O U A A I O X I N E G M A T U Y
V A C C I N E S G I J E U F B L E P A
A C Y T C O L O G N H X R D I T W A G
M B G T E F N M A N T A T S N Y S T T
I M M U N E S Y S T E M I E A H X H P
G P U Y D V A C C U P I L Z N N C O H
R A R U O W W E R R O N M X T M V L A
A T T I T I T E R T I A N C E I T O G
N H I O O M M U T I Y T B V X G O G L
S L K J X E D Y U I D I E T A R X Y J
W O U H I S D G H J K O V R M A I I C
F Z O O N O T I C T U N Z O O I N S K
V B N M S C Y T P O I G V A C C W O U
```

Chapter 12 Pathology, Response to Disease, and Preventive Medicine

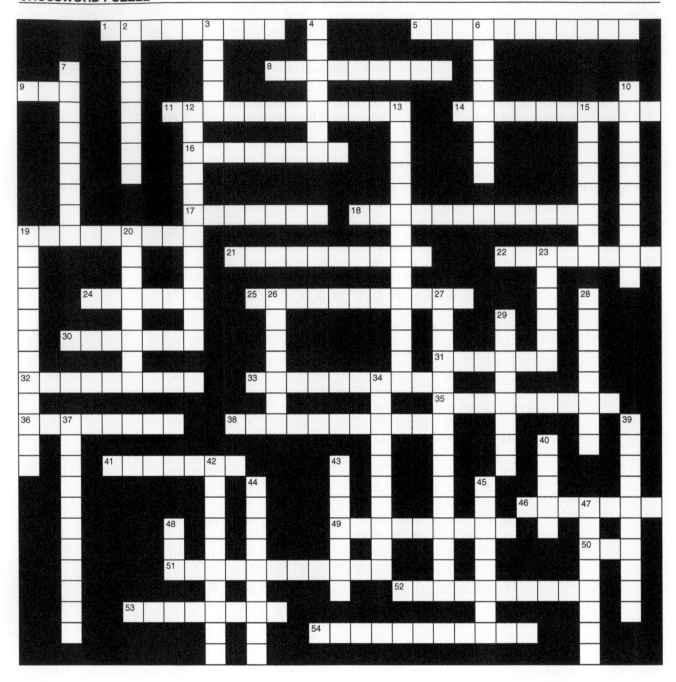

Across

1 The location in which a pathogenic agent is maintained prior to transmission. (9)
5 A severe hypersensitivity reaction. (11)
8 A white blood cell. (9)
9 The primary immunoglobulin associated with allergic and parasitic reactions. (3)
11 The process of coating of the outer surface of pathogens by antibodies to allow easier phagocytosis by macrophages. (12)

Down

2 A normal level of animal disease over time in a given geographic area. (8)
3 A/an __ is an extremely small, nonliving infectious agent, ranging from 30 to 450 nm in diameter, that can cause disease in a wide variety of animals. (5)
4 The visible product of the inflammatory process; usually composed of cellular debris, fluids, and cells that are deposited in tissues and on tissue surfaces. (7)
6 An infectious organism that can cause disease in a host. (8)

Across

14 The cell of the inflammatory system with reddish-orange staining granules that is associated with parasitic infestations and allergic reactions. (10)

16 An antigen that evokes an allergic or hypersensitivity reaction. (8)

17 The type of exudate formed when a purulent material changes into a thick, pasty material. (7)

18 The sanitizing agent found in products such as laundry bleach, which has a wide spectrum of antimicrobial activity. (12)

19 The housing, diet, and environment of animals. (9)

21 Antigens found on the surface of red blood cells that characterize the blood as being a certain type are __ antigens. (2 words) (10)

22 A scar. (8)

24 A/an __ exudate consists primarily of fluid with low protein content. (6)

25 A vaccine that contains whole killed pathogens or selected antigenic subunits in amounts sufficient to induce immunity. (11)

30 Being free from infection. (7)

31 A/an __ is inactivated antigenic toxin molecules that stimulate development of the animal's own antibodies. (6)

32 An organism whose cells have a membrane-bound nucleus. (9)

33 The formation of excessive granulation tissue is described as __ __. (2 words) (10)

35 A chemical substance that causes disease; produced in the cell walls of Gram-negative bacteria and often stimulating the release of pyrogens by the host's cells. (9)

36 The type of cytokine produced by macrophages. (8)

38 The type of lymphocyte that binds to the antigen on a macrophage surface, then secretes specific cytokines to activate other elements of cell-mediated immunity. (2 words) (11)

41 The particular part of the antigen that binds the antibody. (7)

46 A normal level of human disease over time in a given geographic area. (7)

49 An increase over the normal expected number of animal disease cases in a geographic area or over a certain time period. (9)

50 The second most common antibody in blood; the major immunoglobulin isotype produced in a primary immune response. (3)

51 __ tissue is the highly vascularized connective tissue produced after extensive tissue damage. (11)

52 After a monocyte leaves the bloodstream and enters tissue at the site of inflammation, it becomes an activated __. (10)

53 __ bacteria cause the host to produce a suppurative exudate. (8)

54 Type of lymphocyte that can be transformed into plasma cells upon antigenic stimulation, to produce antibodies. (11)

Down

7 Rupture of a red blood cell membrane. (9)

10 The process by which cells exit the blood vessels by squeezing through the microscopic space between the endothelial cells lining the blood vessels. (10)

12 Ingestion of substances by cells. (12)

13 An exudate composed primarily of lymphocytes and monocytes is said to be __. (14)

15 Suppurative exudates are also known as __ exudates. (8)

19 An increase above the body's normal temperature due to such things as drugs, toxins, or external temperatures. (12)

20 A postmortem examination of an animal body. (8)

23 The protein coat that surrounds the genetic material of viruses. (6)

26 The type of immunity conferred to the body by exposure to a pathogen by natural means rather than through vaccination. (7)

27 The term used to characterize pathogens, especially viruses that infect epithelial cells such as respiratory, intestinal, or urinary epithelium. (15)

28 An injury whereby the epithelium is removed from the tissue surface. (8)

29 A chemical substance that causes disease; often produced by Gram-positive bacteria and secreted into the surrounding medium. (8)

34 A tear or jagged wound. (10)

37 The term used to characterize pathogens, especially viruses that infect cells of the central nervous system. (11)

39 A humoral or cell-mediated immune response against antigens found in a body's own cells. (10)

40 An injury caused by physical means, with disruption of normal structures. (5)

42 The cell into which a B lymphocyte is transformed to produce and secrete antibodies. (2 words) (10)

43 Another name for a fever. (7)

44 A bruise or injury with no break in the surface of the tissue. (9)

45 The study of the causes of disease. (8)

47 An increase over the normal expected number of human disease cases in a geographic area or over a certain time period. (8)

48 The most common antibody, found in the highest concentration in blood. (3)

13 Management of Wounds, Fractures, and Other Injuries

LEARNING OBJECTIVES

After reviewing this chapter, the reader will be able to:
- Describe the phases of wound healing
- Identify the categories of wounds
- Explain the principles of first-aid treatment of wounds
- Explain the principles of wound closure
- Give examples of the types and application of bandages
- Give examples of the types and application of splints and casts
- Distinguish ways in which specific types of wounds are managed

DEFINITIONS

Define the following.

1. Abrasion:

_____

_____

2. Acute wound:

_____

_____

3. Contamination:

_____

_____

4. Debridement:

_____

_____

5. Epinephrine:

_____

_____

6. Epithelialization:

_____

_____

7. Exudate:

_____

_____

8. Infection:

_____

_____

9. Nonchemical debridement:

_____

_____

10. Vasoconstriction:

_____

_____

MATCHING

_____ 1. Carpal flexion sling

_____ 2. Ehmer sling

_____ 3. External coaptation

_____ 4. Nonadherent dressing

_____ 5. Occulsive dressing

_____ 6. Robert Jones bandage

_____ 7. Semipermeable dressing

_____ 8. Velpeau sling

A. Configures to hold the carpus in flexion, thus reducing tension on the flexor surface.

B. Placed to keep weight-bearing off the coxofemoral joint.

C. Placed to hold the forelimb against the chest and prevent weight-bearing of the limb.

D. When used on a wound, this allows for air transfer but not fluid transfer.

E. After orthopedic surgery on a rear limb, this is placed to help protect the limb initially.

F. A granulating wound needs this placed to keep it from sticking to the wound.

G. Using this requires less changing and accelerates epithelialization compared to an exposed wound.

H. This is used on the outside of a limb to join or maintain two ends together such as a broken bone or cut tendon.

MUTIPLE CHOICE

There is only one most correct answer for each question.

1. The process of wound healing:
   a. is a simple biologic event that is well understood
   b. is regulated at the molecular level and is well understood
   c. is described in three phases: inflammatory, repair, and maturation
   d. is a dynamic process and more than one phase is occurring at a time

2. Which of the following is not true?
   a. Old animals heal slowly.
   b. Malnourished animals heal slowly.
   c. Sharp surgical incision causes slower healing.
   d. Corticosteroids cause slower healing.

3. Which of the following about wound lavage is not true?
   a. It is necessary to remove debris and loose particles.
   b. It reduces the number of bacteria in the wound.
   c. It can be done before any sampling of the wound for culture.
   d. It should be performed with a warm, sterile, balanced solution.

4. Lavage is accomplished mostly by mechanical action. This is performed by using a:
   a. 35-ml syringe and high pressure
   b. 35-ml syringe and moderate pressure
   c. 60-ml syringe and high pressure
   d. 60-ml syringe and moderate pressure

5. Wound closure is performed using one of four methods based on the nature of the wound. The four methods are:
   a. primary wound closure, first-intention healing, appositional healing, delayed primary closure.
   b. first-intention healing, appositional healing, delayed primary closure, second-intention healing.
   c. primary wound healing, delayed primary closure, second-intention healing, third-intention healing.
   d. first-intention healing, delayed primary closure, second-intention healing, third-intention healing.

6. An abscess is considered what type of wound?
   a. clean, sharply incised
   b. mildly contaminated
   c. significantly contaminated
   d. granulation tissue

7. Bandages are considered helpful in all the following except:
   a. as a type of primary wound healing
   b. protecting the wound from additional trauma/contamination
   c. preventing hematoma formation
   d. as a form of debriding a wound

8. Diphenhydramine is usually given as a pretreatment for this type of wound:
   a. gunshot
   b. snakebite
   c. burns
   d. bite wounds

9. Decubital ulcers generally are found in which patient?
   a. trauma patient
   b. newborn patient
   c. postsurgical, young patient
   d. recumbent patient

10. Which of the following is not common practice for recumbent patients:
    a. Change patient position frequently.
    b. Keep the skin clean and moist.
    c. Provide sufficient soft padding.
    d. Provide a well-balanced, high-protein diet.

1. How does a wound get created?

_____

_____

_____

_____

2. List the seven factors to consider when determining the type of wound closure to be used.

1. _____

2. _____

3. _____

4. _____

5. _____

6. _____

7. _____

3. Describe wet-to-wet and wet-to-dry bandaging.

_____

_____

_____

_____

4. List the indications for drain placement.

_____

_____

_____

_____

5. List the steps for standard application of any bandage to a limb.

_____

_____

_____

_____

6. Describe the three types of thermal burns.

_____

_____

_____

_____

_____
_____
_____
_____

TRUE OR FALSE

1. _____ Pressure sores and vascular ulcers are types of chronic wounds.

2. _____ The phases of wound healing occur in this order: debridement, inflammation, repair, maturation.

3. _____ Infection and corticosteroids delay or stop wound repair.

4. _____ Contaminated tissue becomes infected if the bacteria multiply to a critical number of organisms per gram of tissue and then invade the tissue.

5. _____ Third intention healing is where large or grossly contaminated wounds are allowed to heal completely without any surgery.

6. _____ Application of topical medications to aid in wound healing is recommended.

7. _____ Occlusive bandages are preferred when bandaging an injury in the field or before transport.

8. _____ Drains are used in wounds to help decrease the formation of tissue pockets and dead space.

9. _____ Formation of excess granulation tissue during wound healing is common in dogs.

10. _____ Closure of decubital ulcers is usually very successful.

11. _____ Puncture wounds usually are small holes with extensive deep tissue damage and contain foreign material and bacteria deep in the wound.

12. _____ Arrows can be removed by the client to help with transport to the hospital.

13. _____ Burn wounds normally can be managed by primary closure.

14. _____ Splints and casts should be checked daily in hospital and weekly once an animal has been sent home.

15. _____ In a modified Thomas splint, the traction should be significant within the splint, so as not to create excessive pressure.

MATCHING

Match which layer the following bandage material may be used in (some can be in more than one layer).

Possible layers of a bandage

_____ 1. Primary layer

_____ 2. Secondary layer

_____ 3. Tertiary layer

Bandage Material
A. Stirrups
B. Cast padding
C. Cling gauze
D. Vet Wrap
E. Elasticon

Chapter 13   Management of Wounds, Fractures, and Other Injuries

Answer each of the following questions by writing the answers on the corresponding lines below. The letters in boxes will form the answer to the Super Clue.

1. This is also known as healing by contraction and epithelialization, then suturing.

2. This apparatus prevents quadriceps contracture after distal femoral fracture repair in young animals.

3. This phase of wound healing can be performed by a veterinarian or the animal's own body will try to do it in the form of an eschar.

4. This provides a simple conduit for gravity flow and is made out of soft latex rubber.

5. This device is used most frequently to provide maximum support/immobilization externally.

6. This is the most commonly used bandage for temporary immobilization of fractures distal to the elbow or stifle before surgery.

7. This causes vasoconstriction and helps reduce hemorrhage when added to local anesthetics.

8. These medications should not be added to wound lavage fluids.

9. This can happen to the incision if the wound is closed prematurely.

10. This phase of wound healing may last for several years.

11. This is another name for primary wound closure.

12. These is another name for second-intention healing.

13. These synthetic hormones depress all phases of wound healing.

14. This layer of bandaging comes in contact with the wound itself.

15. This is the most frequently used material for casts today.

16. This type of wound heals by reepithelialization and is a partial-thickness injury of the epidermis that exposes the deep dermis.

17. This is another name for skin maceration in horses.

Super Clue: This apparatus helps to prevent animals from chewing their bandages and also prevents them from injuring their eyes, ears, or any other part of the head.

1. __ __ __ __ __ __ __ ☐ __ __ __ __ __ __ __ __ __ __ __

2. __ __ __ __ __ __ ☐ __ __ __ __ __ __ __ __ __

3. __ __ __ __ __ __ __ __ ☐ __ __ __

4. __ __ ☐ __ __ __ __ __ __

5. __ ☐ __ __

6. __ __ ☐ __ __ __ __ __ __ __

7. __ __ __ __ ☐ __ __ __ __ __

8. __ __ __ __ __ __ ☐ __ __ __

9. __ __ ☐ __ __ __ __ __ __

10. __ __ __ __ __ ☐ __ __ __ __

11. __ __ __ __ __ __ __ __ ☐ __ __

12. __ __ __ ☐ __ __ __ __ __

13. _ _ _ _ _ _ ☐ _ _ _ _ _ _ _ _

14. _ _ _ _ _ _ _ ☐ _ _ _ _

15. _ _ ☐ _ _ _

16. _ _ _ _ _ ☐ _ _ _

17. _ _ _ _ _ _ ☐ _ _ _

WORD SEARCH

Identify the term described then find the words in the Word Search below.

1. This type of splint helps immobilize the elbow or shoulder by extending over the trunk _____

2. This sling prevents weight-bearing on the forelimb _____

3. This type of gun produces what is considered a low-velocity projectile _____

4. This is used to treat snakebites _____

5. This burn is caused by exposure to excessive heat _____

6. In terms of degrees of burn this type does not cause any blisters or vesicles to form in animals (it does in people)

   _____

7. This is the term given to the dark brown, insensitive, leathery covering produced by a third-degree burn

   _____

8. This type of burn can cause acute pulmonary edema _____

9. This is a type of bite wound _____

10. A bandage in this shape is used to help treat decubital ulcers _____

X	A	N	T	I	V	E	N	I	N	B	A	H	E	P
E	L	E	C	T	R	I	C	A	L	C	O	L	N	U
S	E	A	H	S	E	C	N	H	A	N	D	G	U	N
C	P	B	E	M	F	T	H	E	R	M	A	L	G	C
H	J	I	E	A	U	I	A	H	R	E	N	O	T	T
A	N	T	C	P	U	N	R	V	E	L	P	E	A	U
R	O	T	R	A	N	B	L	S	H	E	U	L	N	R
X	N	I	A	F	D	O	N	U	T	A	N	T	I	E

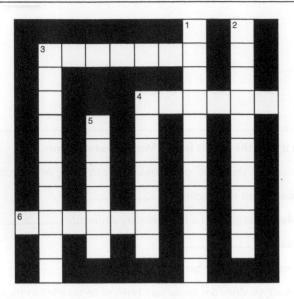

Across

3 A soft rubber tube that is surgically placed in a wound to drain fluid is a ___ drain. (7)

4 The type of adhesive tape that allows evaporation of fluid from the bandage and allows movement of fluid into the wound. (6)

6 The ___ healing phage is characterized by blood vessel formation, collagen deposition, granulation tissue formation, epithelialization, and wound contraction. (6)

Down

1 The ___ healing phase occurs when neutrophils enter the wound to scavenge debris and kill bacteria to decontaminate it. (11)

2 The ___ healing phase occurs when collagen is remodeled and realigned along tension lines and cells that are no longer needed are removed. (10)

3 The excess granulation tissue that may form on a horse's leg. (2 words) (10)

4 First-intention healing is also called ___ healing. (7)

5 Layers of necrotic tissues that slough off. (6)

14 Anesthesia, Analgesia, and Anesthetic Nursing

LEARNING OBJECTIVES

After reviewing this chapter, the reader will be able to:
- Define the role of veterinary technicians in anesthesia and perioperative pain management
- State the significance of and methods for managing perioperative pain
- Identify the goals and fundamentals of anesthesia
- Compare and contrast the types of anesthetic agents, their effects, and their advantages and disadvantages, used in the anesthetic induction and maintenance of small animals
- Outline the equipment used for anesthetizing animals, be able to identify the function and use of each component of the anesthetic machine, and differentiate between rebreathing and nonrebreathing circuits, a precision and nonprecision vaporizer, and a VOC and VIC
- Describe the rationale for each of the anesthetic machine components and its use
- Prepare and maintain anesthetic machines and the associated equipment
- List and describe the steps involved in anesthetizing animals for induction
- Explain the procedures used in medicating and monitoring animals before, during, and after anesthesia
- Prepare a small animal patient, anesthetic equipment, anesthetic agents, and accessories for general anesthesia
- Discuss endotracheal intubation including its advantages and potential complications
- State the standards for providing for patient positioning, comfort, and safety during anesthetic maintenance
- List factors that affect patient recovery from anesthesia, the signs of recovery, and appropriate monitoring during recovery

FILL IN THE BLANK

1. A growing concern in veterinary medicine is _____ control, pre-, peri- and postoperative.

2. It is very helpful to know the normal behavior of the _____ when assessing it for pain.

3. It has been demonstrated that pain is more easily managed if analgesics are given _____ before a patient experiences pain.

4. Using several analgesic drugs, each with a different mechanism of action, is called _____ therapy.

5. Tranquilizers and sedatives are typically used as _____ medications to calm the patient and reduce the amount of anesthetic needed.

6. Analgesic agents are needed to suppress the _____ pain mechanisms that remain active during anesthesia.

7. The process by which pain information is carried from the periphery sense receptors in the skin and the viscera to the cerebral cortex through network of neuronal relays is called _____.

8. The most important step in an anesthetic procedure is the _____ _____ because all anesthetic decisions are based on health status.

9. Standard practice is to withhold food for _____ to _____ hours and water for _____ to _____ hours before anesthetic induction.

10. In high-volume clinics, when several people are involved in patient evaluation and preparation, _____

   _____ should be completed before any anesthetic procedure is done to ensure that appropriate items are available, important health issues have been addressed, and all involved persons have been informed.

11. Administration of the induction agent transitions the patient to unconsciousness. When jaw muscle tone and

   _____ reflexes are lost, intubate the patient.

12. Applying _____ to the larynx by spray or with a cotton-tipped swab, especially in cats and swine, facilitates intubation.

13. For most procedures and patients the flowmeter is set to deliver _____ L/min of oxygen, and the

    vaporizer is set to deliver a concentration of _____ to _____ percent.

14. If anesthetic administration is not reduced in the presence of _____ or _____, patients may become too deeply anesthetized, with further compromise of tissue perfusion.

15. For inhalant agents, potency is determined largely by the lipid solubility of the agent and is reflected by the

    _____ _____ _____.

16. Monitoring should be _____, and data should be recorded every _____ to _____ minutes or when significant changes occur.

17. Flow rates for nonrebreathing systems are high because it is the only way CO_2 is flushed away from the patient; flow

    rates of _____ to _____ ml/kg/min or 2 to 3 times the minute ventilation are recommended.

18. Maintenance flow rate for a rebreathing circuit operated as a closed system is equal to the patient's calculated oxygen

    consumption rate of _____.

19. The primary means of increasing _____ uptake is to increase the vaporizer setting.

20. Monitoring a patient under anesthesia primarily focuses on the _____ and _____ systems.

21. An SpO_2 reading of _____ % is needed before visible cyanosis occurs in a patient.

22. When the peripheral pulse rate is less than the heart rate it is referred to as a _____ _____.

23. Pulse deficits occurring at a rate of _____/_____ heartbeats (10%) or more may significantly diminish coronary and peripheral perfusion and require immediate attention.

24. Hemoglobin has _____ times the affinity for carbon monoxide than oxygen, and its presence reduces the oxygen-transporting capability of hemoglobin, resulting in hypoxemia.

25. Capillary refill time (CRT) of less than _____ seconds in small animals and less than _____ seconds in large animals is considered normal.

26. Anesthetics produce dose-dependent decreases in blood pressure; therefore, monitoring blood pressure during

    anesthesia is useful for _____ determination and evaluation of patient health status.

SHORT ANSWER

1. When is anesthesia or sedation needed in the veterinary setting?

   _____

   _____

   _____

   _____

2. Define pain.

   _____

   _____

   _____

3. Drugs utilized for analgesia cause various dose-dependent effects; give these for Opioids:

_____

_____

Nonsteroidal antiinflammatory drugs (NSAIDs):

_____

_____

4. The goals of every anesthetic-analgesic plan are to predict, prevent, recognize, and correct complications. Complications can be prevented by:

_____

_____

5. List six of the physical signs of pain.

1. _____

2. _____

3. _____

4. _____

5. _____

6. _____

6. Patient characteristics such as species, breed, age, and gender may prompt special considerations. List some of these known characteristics for each of the four groups listed below.

Sight hounds

_____

_____

_____

Brachycephalic breeds

_____

_____

_____

Pediatric patients

_____

_____

_____

Geriatric patients

_____

_____

_____

7. Describe how to check the anesthetic machine out for a day's worth of work.

Checklist for Daily Inspection of Anesthetic Equipment

_____

_____

_____

_____

_____

_____

_____

_____

8. Give the appropriate fluid delivery set for each of these animals:

a. 6-kg Mini-Dachshund

_____

b. 30-kg Labrador Retriever

_____

c. 50-kg Mastiff

_____

9. Why should an endotracheal tube be lubricated before insertion?

_____

_____

10. How do you check the endotracheal tube for correct placement inside the animal?

_____

_____

_____

11. Explain how inhalant anesthetics work in the body from first inhalation to death.

_____

_____

_____

_____

12. What are the advantages and disadvantages of using inhalant gas anesthetic?

_____

_____

_____

_____

13. How often throughout the maintenance period should a patient be ventilated, and at what pressure?

_____

_____

_____

_____

14. Define:
    Anesthetic uptake

_____

_____

    Anesthetic distribution

_____

_____

    Tissue uptake

_____

_____

    Anesthetic elimination

_____

_____

15. Explain why a fat animal's recovery is often longer than that of a thin animal.

_____

_____

_____

_____

16. Explain why it is so important to use a monitoring chart and to be diligent in monitoring a patient.

_____

_____

_____

_____

Chapter 14 Anesthesia, Analgesia, and Anesthetic Nursing

17. Describe how to monitor respiration during an anesthetic procedure.

_____

_____

_____

_____

18. Describe how to monitor the cardiovascular function during an anesthetic procedure.

_____

_____

19. Describe what each of the listed monitoring devices, methods of observation, or measurements used during an anesthetic procedure reveal about the condition of the patient.

Stethoscope

_____

_____

_____

Esophageal stethoscope

_____

_____

_____

Electrocardiograph

_____

_____

_____

Pulse oximeter

_____

_____

_____

Apnea monitor

_____

_____

_____

Ultrasonic Doppler

_____

_____

_____

Oscillometric method

_____

_____

_____

Capnometer

_____

_____

_____

Central venous pressure

_____

_____

_____

20. When should the endotracheal tube be removed from a recovering patient?

_____

_____

_____

_____

WORD SEARCH

Identify the term described and then find the words in the Word Search.

1. A mild to profound degree of CNS depression in which the patient is drowsy but may be aroused by painful stimuli

   _____

2. A chemical substance that can combine with a cell receptor and cause a reaction or create an active site

   _____

3. The narrowing of the blood vessels resulting from contraction of the muscular wall of the vessels, particularly the

   large arteries, small arterioles, and veins _____

4. A pressure gauge for comparing pressures of a gas _____

5. Is measured as the frequency of breathing multiplied by the volume of each breath. It maintains normal concentrations
   of oxygen and carbon dioxide in the alveolar gas and, through the process of diffusion, also maintains normal partial

   pressures of oxygen and carbon dioxide in the blood flowing from the capillaries _____

6. The inability to feel pain while still conscious _____

7. A drug that produces numbness or stupor _____

8. A device used to measure blood pressure _____

9. Loss of feeling or awareness _____

10. The neural processes of encoding and processing noxious stimuli _____

11. The pressure of blood in the artery when the heart contracts _____

12. A drug or other chemical substance capable of reducing the physiologic activity of another chemical substance

    _____

13. An instrument that measures the oxygen in arterial blood _____

14. The action of certain medications that inhibit the transmission of parasympathetic nerve impulses and thereby reduce spasms of smooth muscle (such as that, for example, in the bladder) _____

15. An unpleasant sensory or emotional experience associated with actual or potential tissue damage _____

16. Transient cessation of respiration _____

17. The rate at which the heart beats _____

18. Any disturbance of the heart's rhythm resulting in fewer than normal heartbeats _____

19. The transport of oxygen from the outside air to the cells within tissues, and the transport of carbon dioxide in the opposite direction _____

20. Excessive slowness in the action of the heart _____

21. An instrument used to measure the carbon dioxide (CO_2) concentration in an air sample _____

22. Pressure of blood in the artery when the heart relaxes between beats _____

23. Ultrasound device that a technician may use to sense the presence or absence of flow in blood vessels _____

24. Abnormally rapid beating of the heart _____

25. Kind of stethoscope placed during anesthesia at the level of the heart to amplify the heartbeat, audible from a distance _____

26. The lung volume representing the normal volume of air displaced between normal inspiration and expiration when extra effort is not applied _____

27. Part of the anesthetic machine that receives medical gases from the pressure regulator _____

28. Reduced rate and depth of ventilation as determined by increased arterial carbon dioxide levels above 45 mm Hg _____

29. The process of administration of a series of bolus injections and discontinuing them when the desired depth is reached _____

30. A state of relaxation and calmness characterized by a lack of anxiety or concern without significant drowsiness _____

31. A medical instrument that is used to obtain a view of the vocal folds and the glottis, which is the space between the cords _____

```
C B J R N J Z R X S N E G C J S H P V N R X N G F
F I B Q G A M E E Q S I E I P N X B O D Z F L L B
B L G V O I R D B O R U L H R P F I Q N P T Z B P
H R G R H A A C P K E T Y E R I T N G I W V C A M
Y Z A W E T D H O A Z G Z Q H A E O X E Q R R B A
P A Q D Y N A Z C T M X W D Z T I T R A T I O N I
E E N O Y G I K N O T T C I R T S N O C O S A V M
R T N T E C P L M P N C L G W D G O L N G K L X H
C O S A A B A A O O H I F Q V O B G V H Z P E W T
A X L I I G N R C H U L A R Y N G O S C O P E P Y
P I E Z N O O I D Q C Z Y I A N E S T H E S I A H
N M R C M O C N N I W I R H D B U U Y N R C R S R
I E D E R E G A I F A Y T Y T R P E O H V A E E R
A T T L P W R A X S L P C N V H A I W R S P L M A
E E A T E T L P L H T I L I A H T C E R P N P U Y
R R I N O I T A R I P S E R L A R T Y R Y O P L D
B O C I L O T S Y S A O N Q L O E N S H T G O O A
N E P Y A O W Y P E H V Z I A M T N T T C R D V R
O S Z Q I N P D N C R Y T Q O C E S O X G A E L B
P U L S E Q W P D H F N O N W Y M P A U O P T A F
A I S E G L A N A H E A A K Z B W Q A I Z H I D E
B U E F M W V L J V X M D U V F O L K I D O M I G
E Y O U S G G B J K T X T P F Q L J N J N Q J T R
O I W X C I E F S A O X K D C V F G U T C X R X T
Z K U Y Y J R E X Q R A C D J V H A J V P Q F L L
```

155

155

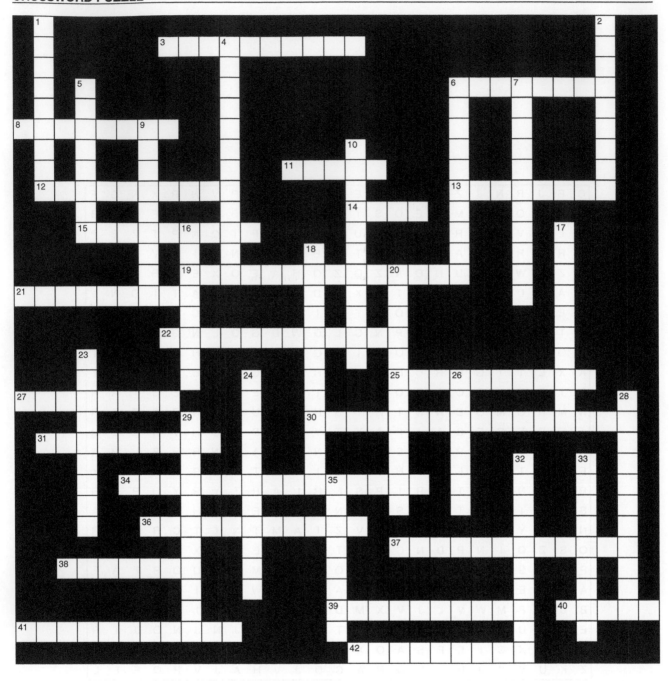

Across

3 __ therapy is the use of several analgesic drugs, each with a different mechanism of action, resulting in lower dosages and increased safety for the animal. (10)

6 __ blood pressure is the pressure of blood in the artery when the heart contracts. (8)

8 Segmental or __ anesthesia is achieved by blocking the nerve or nerves that supply a segment of the body. (8)

11 A/an __ monitor is a sensor to determine whether a patient is breathing. (5)

12 A drug given to prevent vomiting. (10)

13 Unconsciousness induced by a narcotic drug. (8)

14 An unpleasant sensory or emotional experience associated with actual or potential tissue damage. (4)

15 The __ bag is a rebreathing bag that provides a gas volume sufficient for the patient to inhale maximally without creating negative pressure in the circuit. (9)

19 Anesthetic breathing circuits in which exhaled gases are discharged to the environment and do not pass back to the patient. (14)

21 The inability to feel pain while still conscious. (9)

22 A medical instrument used to view the vocal folds and glottis. (12)

25 Loss of feeling or awareness. (10)

27 A muscular disease in which the muscle fibers do not function for any one of many reasons, resulting in muscular weakness. (8)

30 A device used to measure blood pressure. (16)

31 Passage of oxygenated blood through body tissues. (9)

34 The action of certain medications that inhibit the transmission of parasympathetic nerve impulses and thereby reduce spasms of smooth muscle. (15)

36 Failure of full expansion of the lung. (11)

37 An instrument for measuring the changes in pulsations in the arteries of the extremities. (12)

38 A pulse __ is the difference between the heart rate and the pulse rate, as in atrial fibrillation. (7)

39 A drug or other chemical substance capable of reducing the physiologic activity of another chemical substance. (10)

40 The lung volume representing the normal volume of air displaced between normal inspiration and expiration when extra effort is not applied. (5)

41 Excess carbon dioxide in the blood. (11)

42 The part of the anesthetic machine that receives medical gases from the pressure regulator. (9)

Down

1 A deficiency in the amount of oxygen reaching body tissues. (9)

2 A brief, involuntary twitching of a muscle or a group of muscles. (9)

4 The conversion of pain stimuli into electrical impulses. (12)

5 A pulse __ is a device that detects changes in oxygen saturation of hemoglobin by calculating the difference between levels of oxygenated and deoxygenated blood. (8)

6 The __ system is the part of the anesthetic machine attached to the exhaust valve that collects waste gases and directs them out of the building or into a charcoal canister. (10)

7 An abnormally rapidly beating heart. (11)

9 Information gained from the patient and others regarding the patient's medical history. (9)

10 The transport of oxygen from the outside air to the cells within tissues, and the transport of carbon dioxide in the opposite direction. (11)

16 The central venous pressure describes the pressure of blood in the thoracic __ __ near the right atrium of the heart. (2 words) (8)

17 __ analgesia refers to taking steps to predict and prevent pain before it occurs. (10)

18 The movement of an electrical impulse along a peripheral nerve to the spinal cord and brain. (12)

20 Primary __ describes pain sensitivity that occurs directly in the damaged tissues. (12)

23 A component of the anesthetic machine that produces a controlled and predictable concentration of anesthetic vapor in the carrier gas by delivering a diluted anesthetic to the patient. (9)

24 An esophageal __ is an instrument placed in the esophagus during anesthesia at the level of the heart to amplify the heartbeat. (11)

26 __ pain is well-localized pain that results from the activation of peripheral nociceptors without injury to the peripheral nerve or central nervous system. (7)

28 Excessive slowness in the action of the heart. (11)

29 The afferent activity produced in the peripheral and central nervous system by stimuli that have the potential to damage tissue, initiated by pain receptors. (11)

32 A device that determines respiratory rate and the end tidal CO_2 by estimating partial CO_2 in the bloodstream at the end of expiration, when CO_2 levels of the expired gas are approximately equal to alveolar and arterial CO_2 ($PaCO_2$). (10)

33 The __ blood pressure is the pressure of blood in the artery when the heart relaxes between beats. (9)

35 A form of regional anesthesia involving injection of drugs through a catheter placed into the subarachnoid space of the spinal cord. (8)

15 Principles of Surgical Nursing

LEARNING OBJECTIVES

After reviewing this chapter, the reader will be able to:
- Describe and explain surgical terminology
- Discuss principles of aseptic technique
- Give examples of methods used to disinfect or sterilize surgical instruments and supplies
- Describe procedures for preparing the surgical site and surgical team
- Identify surgical instruments and explain their uses and maintenance
- Compare and contrast types of suture needles and suture materials

SHORT ANSWER

1. After what length of time are skin sutures typically removed?

_____

2. Other than suture, what might be used for vessel ligation during surgery?

_____

3. What is the most common form of gas sterilization found in the veterinary hospital, and for what equipment is it typically used?

_____

_____

4. Name two accepted methods of performing surgical scrubbing.

_____

_____

5. How are synthetic absorbable suture materials broken down?

_____

6. Why should hair be clipped liberally around the proposed surgical incision?

_____

_____

7. Explain the major function of surgical masks.

_____

_____

8. What might the veterinary technician be responsible for in the postsurgical period?

_____

_____

9. Differentiate between contamination and infection of a wound.

_____

_____

MATCHING

Match the following surgical instruments with their primary function.

_____ 1. Hemostatic forceps

_____ 2. Needle holders

_____ 3. Retractors

_____ 4. Scissors

_____ 5. Scalpels and blades

_____ 6. Tissue forceps

A. Used to incise tissue
B. Used for cutting tissue
C. Grasp and manipulate curved needles
D. Clamp and hold tissue and blood vessels
E. Crushing instrument used to clamp blood vessels
F. Used to retract tissue and improve exposure

Match the following surgical procedures with their definition.

_____ 1. Herniorrhaphy

_____ 2. Orchiectomy

_____ 3. Gastrotomy

_____ 4. Thoracotomy

_____ 5. Enterotomy

_____ 6. Cystotomy

_____ 7. Urethrotomy

_____ 8. Laparotomy

_____ 9. Mastectomy

_____ 10. Onychectomy

A. Incision into the intestine
B. Removal of part or all of one or more mammary glands
C. Incision into the urinary bladder
D. Surgical removal of a claw
E. Incision into a simple stomach
F. Incision into the abdominal cavity
G. Surgical removal of testes
H. Incision into thoracic cavity
I. Surgical repair of abnormal opening
J. Incision into the urethra

Match the following surgical incisions with their location or benefit.

_____ 1. Flank incision

_____ 2. Ventral midline incision

_____ 3. Median sternotomy

_____ 4. Paramedian incision

_____ 5. Paracostal incision

A. Parallel to the last rib
B. Lateral and parallel to the ventral midline
C. Perpendicular to long axis of body, caudal to last rib
D. Offers excellent exposure of entire abdominal cavity
E. Used when all lung fields need to be visualized

FILL IN THE BLANK

1. _____ is the term used to describe all precautions taken to prevent contamination or infection of a surgical wound.

2. Surgical procedures are described using _____ combined with root words.

3. _____ refers to the destruction of all microorganisms (bacteria, viruses, spores) on a surface or object.

4. Hospital-acquired infections are called _____.

5. Surgical mesh may be used to _____ or reinforce traumatized or devitalized tissues.

6. Curved instruments are passed to the surgeon with the _____ side up.

7. _____ ensures that the hand never comes into contact with the outside of the surgical gown or glove.

8. Organic nonabsorbable suture is made of _____ or _____.

9. Surgical instrument manufacturers may recommend rinsing, cleaning, and sterilizing instruments in _____ because tap water contains minerals that cause discoloration and staining.

10. Surgical packs may not be completely sterilized if they are _____ or improperly loaded in the autoclave or gas sterilizer container.

11. Subcutaneous infections frequently progress to _____.

12. Prior to sterilization, surgical drapes are folded so that the _____ can be properly positioned over the surgical site without contaminating the drape.

13. A _____ should be available to place needed supplies and equipment on the instrument table or Mayo stand in an operating room.

14. _____ needles have a sharp tip that pierces and spreads tissue without cutting it.

15. Sterile preparation of the surgical site begins after transportation and _____ of the animal on the operating table.

SHORT ANSWERS

1. Identify the three basic components of a suture needle:

   1. _____
   2. _____
   3. _____

2. What are five possible causes of wound dehiscence?

   1. _____
   2. _____
   3. _____
   4. _____
   5. _____

3. List the four main sources of potential contamination during surgery:

   1. _____
   2. _____
   3. _____
   4. _____

4. The four groups of nonabsorbable suture materials are:

   1. _____
   2. _____
   3. _____
   4. _____

5. List six pieces of surgical attire:

1. _____

2. _____

3. _____

4. _____

5. _____

6. _____

6. Name four indications of infection following surgery:

1. _____

2. _____

3. _____

4. _____

7. Name seven factors that influence the effectiveness of all microbial control methods:

1. _____

2. _____

3. _____

4. _____

5. _____

6. _____

7. _____

IDENTIFICATION

1. What gloving method is seen below? _____

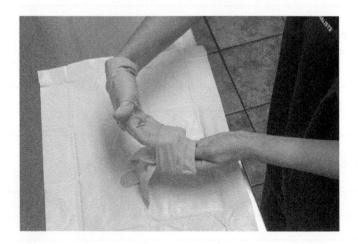

2. What procedure is pictured below? _____

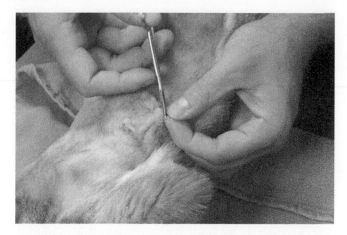

3. What sterilization equipment is seen below? _____

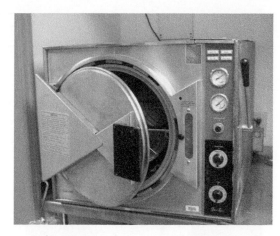

Chapter **15** **Principles of Surgical Nursing**

4. Examples of what type of suture are seen below? _____

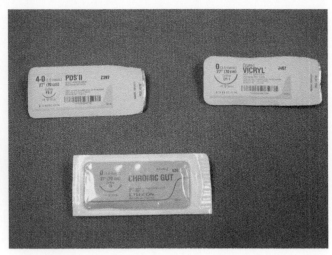

5. Identify both types of sterilization indicator tape seen below:

_____

_____

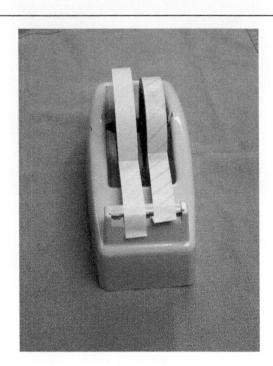

6. What surgical instruments are pictured below?

_____

_____

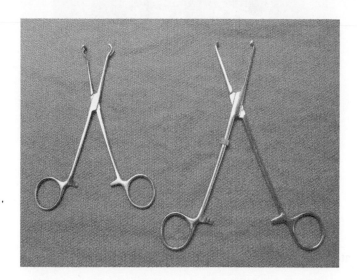

7. What procedure is seen below? _____

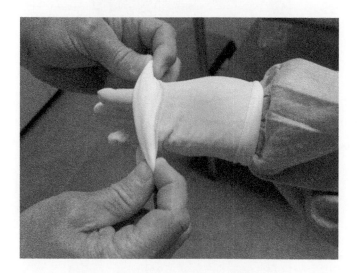

8. The patient seen below is positioned and the field draped for what type of surgery? _____

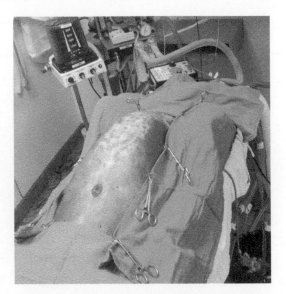

9. What piece of equipment is seen below? _____

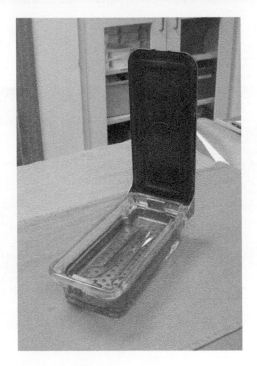

10. What positioning and preparation have been used in the image below?

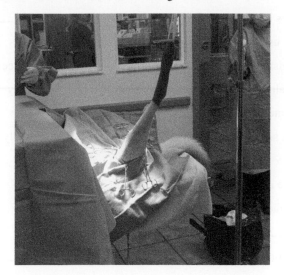

_____

_____

WORD SEARCH

Identify the term described and then find the terms in the Word Search.

1. Infection in the abdominal cavity _____

2. Instrument designed to cut and remove bone pieces _____

3. The presence of microorganisms within or on an object or wound _____

4. Incision into the abdominal cavity, also called celiotomy _____

5. Large crushing instrument used to clamp blood vessels _____

6. Incision into the rumen _____

7. Incision into the thorax _____

8. Surgical removal of the lateral wall of the vertical portion of the external ear canal _____

9. Destruction of most living pathogenic microorganisms on animate (living) objects _____

10. Incision into the abdominal cavity, also called laparotomy _____

11. Instrument designed to bore holes in bone _____

12. Destruction of most pathogenic microorganisms on inanimate objects _____

13. Instrument designed to cut or shape bone and cartilage _____

14. Suture needle used in accessible places where the needle can be manipulated directly with the fingers _____

15. Incision into the urethra _____

16. Delicate scissors designed for fine, precise cuts, often used in ophthalmic procedures _____

17. A sterilization unit that creates high-temperature pressurized steam _____

18. Any strand of material that is used to approximate tissues or ligate blood vessels _____

19. Destruction of all microorganisms (bacteria, viruses, spores) on a surface or object _____

20. A cauterizing needle tip or scalpel generating heat in tissue with a high-frequency current, to provide hemostasis in vessels less than 2 mm in diameter _____

21. Self-retaining retractor with a set screw to maintain tension on tissues, commonly used to retract abdominal wall _____

22. Instrument used to shape bone and cartilage _____

23. Instrument used to scrape surfaces of dense tissue _____

24. Incision into the stomach _____

25. Tissue scissors designed for cutting heavy tissue such as fascia _____

26. Surgical removal of part or all of one or more mammary glands _____

27. Self-retaining retractor with a boxlock to maintain tension on tissues, commonly used in orthopedic surgeries _____

28. Delicate scissors designed for cutting fine, thin tissue _____

29. Microorganisms in the body or a wound multiply and cause harmful effects _____

30. Incision oriented perpendicular to the long axis of the body, caudal to the last rib _____

31. Protrusion of an organ (viscera) through an incision _____

32. Incision into the intestine _____

```
L A S N T N O I T A Z I L I R E T S A C H I S E L
A B E C C P L M E I C V W M K O U L P D E R T N M
P D F N O I S I C N I K N A L F P S R U E G N O R
A W I M N O L B A L F O U R R E T R A C T O R B I
R P A U T O C L A V E Y T E V E D C N P Y T K M C
O L M Q A R O T C A R T E R I P L E G A R C E E N
T B U T M G H J O I K M X E W T O P I T N M L I V
O U P R I N F E C T I O N P I L Q W O E K L E O S
M R N I N S E L D E E N T H G I A R T S L U C T R
Y E O K A U Y S U T U R E K L O M N R A J K T D O
C T I S T D M G R S R O S S I C S S I R I Y R E S
J H T E I E O A Y O P E U A B P E I B A M E O G S
A R C B O M T S H P S M R T S E T T E R U C C A I
G O E I N O O T T A I S K G F D A I S I O M O S C
R T F R P T C R E W X S I V Z J Y P N K L I A T S
E H N T L O A O S Y W I B C E L I O T O M Y G R M
T O I O K E R T M B R S T M S Q D B L U P T U O U
A M S I E T O O Q U S P A E I O N I F E K E L T A
R Y I G I S H M A S T E C T O M Y C R N U Y A O B
E J D N S O T Y V I L S A S T O E A M I H T T M N
C P P A R F A O R T J I E P W D V B M H F R I Y E
S D I E N C P L A S I T I N O T I R E P W D O L Z
I G T P J O L R U M E N O T O M Y S K E I P N I T
V N R L M L O T M T P A Y M O T O C A R O H T F E
E J S N O I T C E S E R R A E L A R E T A L K G M
```

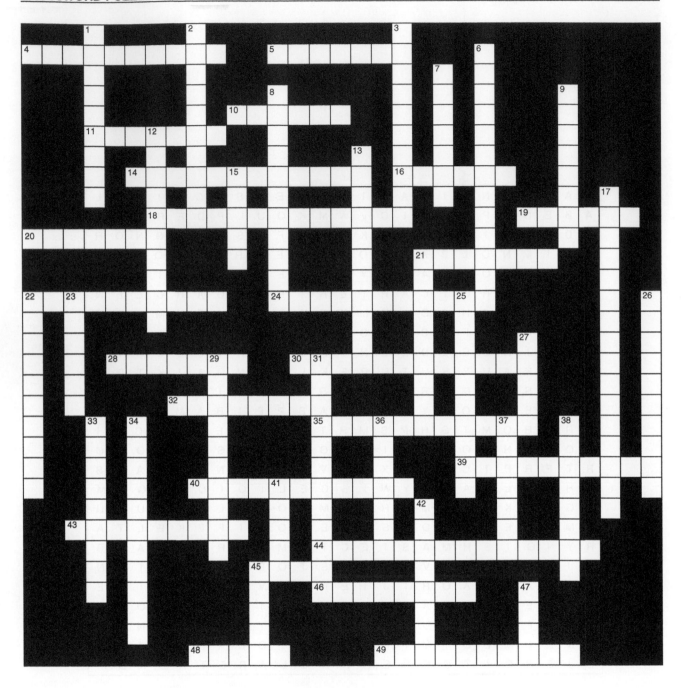

Across

4 The type of needle holders with a ratchet lock just distal to the thumb. (2 words) (10)

5 The self-retaining retractor with a set screw to maintain tension on tissues, commonly used to retract abdominal wall. (7)

10 An instrument used to shape bone and cartilage. (6)

11 The type of suture needle with a sharp tip that pierces and spreads tissues without cutting them. (7)

14 Destruction of most pathogenic microorganisms on inanimate objects. (12)

16 Any strand of material that is used to approximate tissues or ligate blood vessels. (6)

18 The presence of microorganisms within or on an object or wound. (13)

19 An organic nonabsorbable suture material with less tissue reaction than silk but which does not, like cotton, support bacterial growth. (6)

20 A scissors with a blunt tip that can safely be introduced under a dressing for removal. (7)

21 The technique where all precautions are taken to prevent contamination and ultimately infection of a surgical wound. (7)

22 Incision into the stomach. (10)

24 Surgical removal of the testicles. (11)

28 A __ needle is a suture needle with two or three opposing sharp edges, used in tissues that are difficult to penetrate. (7)

30 A castrating instrument to accomplish closed castration, keeping skin intact. (12)

32 A __ section is the surgical removal of newborns via an abdominal incision. (8)

35 Surgical removal of a claw. (11)

39 The type of delicate scissors designed for cutting fine, thin tissue. (10)

40 A castrating instrument to accomplish castration by crushing and severing the spermatic cord. (11)

43 The type of needle holders with a ratchet lock just distal to the thumb, with a blade for cutting suture. (2 words) (9)

44 The process of heating a needle tip or scalpel before it is applied to tissue to provide hemostasis in vessels less than 2 mm in diameter. (14)

45 Another name for a rake retractor is the __ retractor. (4)

46 An instrument designed to bore holes in bone. (8)

48 The type of self-retaining retractor with a boxlock to maintain tension on tissues, commonly used in orthopedic surgeries. (5)

49 Destruction of most living pathogenic microorganisms on animate objects. (10)

Down

1 Another name for a laparotomy. (9)

2 A __ incision is located lateral and parallel to the ventral midline of the animal. (10)

3 The tissue forceps with small serrations on the tips that cause minimal trauma but hold tissue securely. (2 words) (10)

6 Surgical repair of a hernia, by suturing the abnormal opening closed. (13)

7 An instrument used to scrape surfaces of dense tissue. (7)

8 The type of self-retaining retractor with a set screw to maintain tension on tissues, commonly used to retract thoracic wall. (11)

9 The type of small hemostatic forceps with transverse jaw serrations. (8)

12 Protrusion of an organ through an incision. (10)

13 Large crushing instrument used to clamp blood vessels. (11)

15 An incision oriented perpendicular to the long axis of the body, caudal to the last rib. (5)

17 A large crushing forceps often used to control large tissue bundles. (2 words) (16)

21 A sterilization unit that creates high-temperature pressurized steam. (9)

22 Surgical fixation of the stomach to the abdominal wall. (10)

23 __ needles are suture needles that are joined with suture into a continuous unit. (6)

25 Surgical removal of part or all of one or more mammary glands. (10)

26 Incision into the intestine. (10)

27 The type of hemostatic forceps with transverse serrations that extend over only the distal portion of the jaws. (5)

29 The type of infection that is hospital acquired. (10)

31 The type of suture made of a single strand of material. (12)

33 A __ retractor is a self-retaining retractor with a boxlock to maintain tension on tissues, commonly used in neurologic surgeries. (9)

34 The type of needle holders with a spring and latch mechanism for locking. (11)

36 The type of surgical gut that has been exposed to chrome or aldehyde to slow absorption. (7)

37 The type of needle holders with a ratchet lock at the proximal end of the handles of the holder, permitting locking and unlocking simply with a progressive squeezing of the instrument. (7)

38 An instrument designed to cut and remove bone pieces. (8)

41 A type of hemostatic forceps with transverse serrations that extend the entire jaw length. (5)

42 Keith or __ needles are used in accessible places, where the needle can be manipulated directly with the fingers. (8)

45 Plain surgical gut is suture material made from the submucosa of __ intestine or serosa of bovine intestine. (5)

47 The type of delicate scissors designed for fine, precise cuts, often used in ophthalmic procedures. (4)

16 Fluid Therapy and Blood Transfusion

LEARNING OBJECTIVES

After reviewing this chapter, the reader will be able to:

- Explain the distribution of water throughout the body and the differences in the composition of extracellular fluid and intracellular fluid compartments
- Describe how physical exam findings play a role in determining a fluid therapy plan
- Differentiate between crystalloid and artificial colloid solutions
- List and explain indications for fluid therapy
- Identify routes of fluid administration
- Compare the different types of intravenous catheters available and the appropriate use of each
- Explain the physiology of hemostasis and how it relates to a bleeding patient
- Describe the steps necessary in assessing a bleeding patient and identifying the cause of bleeding
- List the types of blood products used in transfusion medicine and give examples of when each product would be used appropriately
- Describe canine and feline blood types
- Distinguish between the information gathered from a blood type compared to a cross-match
- Identify different blood collection methods, giving examples of collection systems available
- Calculate blood product dosages
- Assess patients receiving blood transfusion support
- Identify adverse reactions to blood transfusion

SHORT ANSWER

1. Approximately what percent of lean body mass is composed of fluid, or total body water (TBW)?

_____

2. List the three major fluid compartments that make up TBW.

_____

_____

_____

3. What are some examples of "third space" fluids?

_____

_____

_____

4. What are the major extracellular electrolytes?

_____

_____

_____

5. What are the major intracellular electrolytes? Which is the dominant ion responsible for osmotic pressure?

_____

_____

_____

6. List some common causes of hypokalemia.

_____

_____

_____

7. List some common causes of hyperkalemia.

_____

_____

_____

8. List the three primary systems that help control acid-base balance.

_____

_____

_____

9. What are some important questions to ask clients in regards to their pet's hydration status or history?

_____

_____

_____

10. Which physical examination signs can help estimate hydration status?

_____

_____

_____

TRUE OR FALSE

1. _____ Some extracellular fluids can collect in various parts of the body secondary to infection, injury, or compromised circulation.

2. _____ The movement of solutes across a semipermeable cell membrane from the side with the lower solute concentration to the side with the higher solute concentration until the concentrations equilibrate is called diffusion.

3. _____ Relatively small changes in serum potassium concentration can alter nervous and cardiac functions.

4. _____ The capillary refill time can be an important indication of peripheral perfusion.

5. _____ Skin turgor is the most accurate way to detect or estimate dehydration.

6. _____ Frequent, serial body weight measurement is a good monitoring tool for continued fluid loss during treatment.

7. _____ Dehydration is associated with increases in both PCV and TPP, while PCV reduction alone is seen with splenic contraction.

8. _____ Prothrombin time (PT) measures extrinsic and common clotting pathway activity, whereas activated partial thromboplastin time (aPTT) measures intrinsic and common pathway activity.

9. _____ Fresh-frozen plasma does not contain viable platelets.

10. _____ Dogs differ from cats in that they have significant naturally occurring alloantibodies against the other blood types.

MULTIPLE CHOICE

1. Which of the following is the most abundant and important of the extracellular ions because the distribution of body water is influenced by this electrolyte?
   a. Bicarbonate
   b. Chloride
   c. Sodium
   d. Potassium

2. Clinical signs associated with hypernatremia are usually primarily:
   a. Neurologic in origin
   b. Not detectable
   c. Behavioral
   d. Weight related

3. What is the normal pH of arterial blood?
   a. 7.0
   b. 7.35
   c. 7.4
   d. 7.45

4. Presence of a cardiac murmur may warrant:
   a. Higher fluid rates
   b. Lower fluid rates
   c. Colloid fluid use only
   d. Hypertonic fluid use only

5. A decreasing hematocrit and total plasma protein level suggests:
   a. Dehydration
   b. Infection
   c. Cerebral edema
   d. Hemodilution

6. Which component is critical in maintaining osmotic pressure?
   a. Albumin
   b. Potassium
   c. Sodium
   d. Chloride

Chapter **16** **Fluid Therapy and Blood Transfusion**

7. What is the standard treatment for hypoproteinemia?
   a. Crystalloid fluids
   b. Colloid fluids
   c. Potassium supplementation
   d. Glucose supplementation

8. What is the best test in determining the kidney's ability to concentrate urine?
   a. BUN
   b. Creatinine
   c. Phosphorous
   d. Urine specific gravity

9. Which solutions contain small molecules that, when in solution, can pass through a semipermeable membrane and enter all body compartments?
   a. Natural colloid solutions only
   b. Synthetic colloid solutions only
   c. Crystalloid fluids
   d. Glucose only

10. The ability of a fluid to change the shape of cells by changing their water content is called:
   a. Tonicity
   b. Colloid osmotic pressure
   c. Osmosis
   d. Diffusion

11. Hypertonic solution administration is contraindicated in:
   a. Severe shock
   b. Head trauma
   c. Dehydration
   d. Infection

12. What is a potential complication to synthetic colloid use?
   a. Sepsis
   b. Vomiting
   c. Coagulopathy
   d. Hypothermia

13. What is a useful tool in determining fluid administration rates?
   a. Body temperature
   b. Mentation
   c. Central venous pressure
   d. Body weight

14. Plasma coagulation factors are produced in the:
   a. Kidneys
   b. Spleen
   c. Bone marrow
   d. Liver

15. Which of the following may mask anemia?

    a. Overhydration

    b. Heart murmur

    c. Splenic contraction

    d. Icterus

16. An increased urine specific gravity is most likely to occur in animals with:

    a. Decreased water intake

    b. Increased water intake

    c. IV fluid overload

    d. Hypoproteinemia

MATCHING

Match the blood component listed in Column B with the appropriate recipient in Column A.

Column A

1. _____ A hit-by-car dog: hematocrit 29, total protein 3.0

2. _____ A 17-year-old cat with chronic renal failure: hematocrit 16, total protein 8.0

3. _____ A dog that presents with generalized petechia and ecchymosis: hematocrit 18, total protein 4.0

4. _____ A dog with severe diarrhea; hematocrit is 29, total solids 2.5

5. _____ A suspected Doberman with VWF bleeding from a tooth extraction

Column B

A. Stored whole blood

B. Fresh-frozen plasma

C. Cryoprecipitate

D. RBCs

E. Fresh whole blood

SHORT ANSWER

1. a. What are the advantages of Oxyglobin in trauma?

   b. Why does the hematocrit usually decrease with Oxyglobin use? How can the technician monitor the PCV?

   c. What type of catheter and filter is required for Oxyglobin administration?

2. An anemic, pure-breed British short-hair cat presents to your clinic for a blood transfusion.

   a. How necessary is it to blood type this patient?

   b. The owner declines any blood typing. What are some common signs of a blood transfusion reaction?

   c. List some monitoring techniques necessary during a blood transfusion.

3. a. List the minimum requirements for a canine blood donor.

_____

_____

b. How often can a dog donate blood?

_____

c. What is the minimum (approximate) acceptable hematocrit of the donor dog prior to blood collection?

_____

4. Why are glass collection bottles not currently recommended for blood transfusions?

_____

_____

5. What are the factors to consider when determining how much blood a patient should receive?

_____

_____

_____

6. a. Why is it important to titrate the amount of citrate/anticoagulant needed for a specific amount of blood?

_____

_____

b. What are the signs of citrate toxicity?

_____

_____

c. Are there any tests to confirm citrate toxicity?

_____

_____

d. What is the treatment of citrate toxicity?

_____

_____

7. a. A unit of whole blood taken from the lab refrigerator seems almost black. What could be the reason? Should the blood be used?

_____

_____

b. List the potential ways trauma can be introduced to a unit of red blood cells, creating hemolysis.

_____

_____

_____

Identify the term described and then find the definitions in the Word Search below.

1. pH <7.35 _____

2. pH <7.45 _____

3. Genetically determined markers on the surface of RBC's _____

4. Detection of serological incompatibility _____

5. Movement of solutes _____

6. Mostly interstitial fluid _____

7. Indicated in anemic patients with significant coagulopathy _____

8. Indicated in hypoproteinemic patients _____

9. Solution that shrinks cells _____

10. Common with excessive IV fluids _____

11. Within the cells _____

12. Fluids equaling the sum of sensible and insensible loss _____

13. Concentration of active solutes _____

14. Movement of water _____

15. 60% body weight _____

```
H K T W D X C J M X M K L Z K K C T K W N P L R
R T C G H B N X R L K A I M T J T H F L O V J C
Y M F C W K V V C P C N N K T R K D G X I K G T
Z R Q N F D T X T I K J T H W W O K M N T P Z R
R K X D K Q F F D Z W D R T P O R W T F U D H E
X L C G C V S O B P H K A V L L N K P C L M E T
B Y M T B I S L N M Q L C B W D T P K N O K X A
T V L Y S I Y R L G C Z E P T Z L L M S C T W
O D C O S N V M B R K L L Z M Z R K C X D K R Y
C S M I Y M K M O N O Q L N Q D G T M Z I G A D
B S M N N N X S L H P T U O G L W L X L U V C O
O L J O Z O S D W L T Y L I D G T D L P L T E B
R H O X L M T H D M N T A S M T T D B C F N L L
P N D O A A S R K G R P R U G T J M Q C E G L A
L X H T D E L K E R Z J F F C P L M L P C J U T
X L C T R T R I N P M W L F Y P K F T F N D L O
B H L F L F Y Q T F Y B U I N X R V N T A L A T
M N P N V C J P L Y M H I D H R P J D L N Y R H
Z G N T Z G B K E V J N D N F M K F K Y E T F Q
C K R W N O S M O T I C P R E S S U R E T R L F
N T V Q Q T K J C B L Z T Y Z B C K Q G N P U T
F R E S H F R O Z E N P L A S M A T Y Y I L I K
B S I S O L A K L A R F L W G D W R C T A M D L
Q B N T L L H K V M L L R X B W L P Q X M N L Y
```

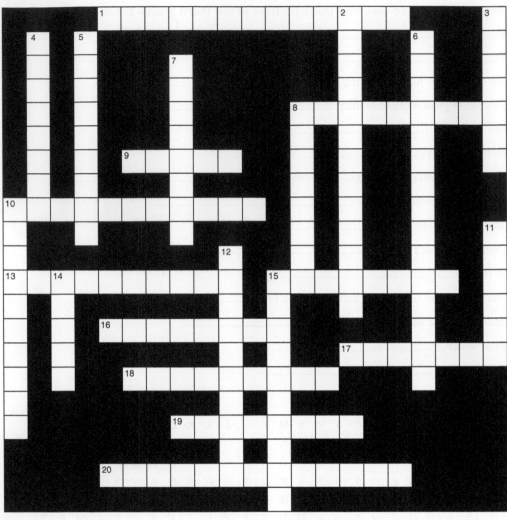

Across

1 An increased concentration of sodium in the blood. (13)

8 A condition in which the blood pH is higher than 7.45. (9)

9 A __ blood crossmatch detects antibodies in the donor plasma against the recipient red blood cells. (5)

10 A decreased concentration of potassium in the blood. (11)

13 The concentration of particles in a solution. (10)

15 A solution that causes cells to neither gain nor lose water. (8)

16 A blood type is a classification of blood based on the presence or absence of inherited __ on the surface of erythrocytes. (8)

17 Fibrin is an insoluble __ that is essential for blood to clot. (7)

18 A solution that causes cells to gain water and swell. (9)

19 Water loss that is easy to measure because it can be seen. (8)

20 Fluid located within cells is called __ fluid. (13)

Down

2 Platelets are irregular, disc-shaped fragments of __ cytoplasm. (13)

3 Movement of water across a semipermeable membrane from the side with high water concentration to low water concentration. (7)

4 The ability of a fluid to change the shape of cells. (8)

5 Movement of molecules across a semipermeable membrane from the side with high concentration of solutes to low concentration of solutes. (9)

6 A precipitate that is prepared from plasma that contains some clotting factors. (15)

7 A/an __ fluid solution is one that is similar in composition to plasma. (8)

8 A condition in which the blood pH is lower than 7.35. (8)

10 Primary __ involves the formation of a platelet plug following injury to a blood vessel. (10)

11 Secondary hemostasis involves the formation of __. (6)

12 A solution that causes cells to lose water. (10)

14 A __ blood crossmatch detects antibodies in the recipient plasma against the donor red blood cells. (5)

15 Water loss that is difficult to measure because it cannot be seen. (10)

180

17 Emergency and Critical Care

LEARNING OBJECTIVES

After reviewing this chapter, the reader will be able to:
- Explain the distribution of water throughout the body and the differences in the composition of extracellular fluid and intracellular fluid compartments
- Describe how physical exam findings play a role in determining a fluid therapy plan
- Differentiate between crystalloid and artificial colloid solutions
- List and explain indications for fluid therapy
- Identify routes of fluid administration
- Compare the different types of intravenous catheters available and the appropriate use of each

MULTIPLE CHOICE

1. Which of the following breathing accessory is not necessary to have in an emergency airway cart?
   a. suction
   b. laryngoscope
   c. heparin flush
   d. endotracheal tubes

2. An AMBU bag is used for which of the following procedures?
   a. intravenous catheter placement
   b. ventilation
   c. nail trim on an aggressive cat
   d. urinary catheter placement

3. During CPR, in the absence of venous access many drugs can be delivered by which route?
   a. intraocular
   b. intratracheal
   c. intramuscular
   d. subcutaneous

4. If a patient presents with an open chest wound, what can the technician do to help stabilize the animal?
   a. Place a generous amount of sterile lube over the wound and apply a sterile dressing.
   b. Obtain a detailed patient history.
   c. Obtain blood and urine samples.
   d. Obtain a TPR.

5. Clinical signs of an immune-mediated blood transfusion reaction include which of the following?
   a. increased appetite
   b. bradycardia
   c. tachycardia
   d. hypothermia

6. Turning a recumbent patient prevents:
   a. bloat
   b. urinary tract infections
   c. atelectasis of the lungs
   d. incisional dehiscence

7. Factors that predispose a patient to a hospital-acquired infection include:
   a. immunosuppression
   b. therapeutic noninvasive procedures
   c. vomiting
   d. frequent walks outside

8. What is the most common complication with rodenticide ingestion?
   a. miosis
   b. muscle tremors
   c. hyperthermia
   d. hemorrhage

9. Excessive furosemide use can lead to:
   a. severe hypokalemia
   b. acidosis
   c. fluid overload
   d. liver failure

10. Dystocia can be characterized by which of the following?
    a. active straining for more than 30 to 60 minutes without delivery of a fetus
    b. excessive vocalization
    c. more than 1 hour between deliveries
    d. excessive vaginal discharge

MATCHING

Match the clinical signs from Column A with the correct disease in Column B.

Column A	Column B
1. _____ Ascites, jugular distension	A. Acute renal failure
2. _____ Lethargy, vomiting, anuria	B. Left-sided congestive heart failure
3. _____ Cough, dyspnea	C. Saddle thrombus
4. _____ Pulselessness, paresis	D. Right-sided congestive heart failure

Match the procedure needed to be performed in Column A with clinical signs in Column B.

Column A	Column B
1. _____ Central venous pressure	A. Muffled heart sounds, poor pulse quality, tachycardia
2. _____ Pericardiocentesis	B. Severe abdominal pain in a patient with pancreatitis
3. _____ Diagnostic peritoneal lavage	C. Pulmonary crackles in a patient in renal failure

SHORT ANSWER

1. List a general protocol for patients with suspected heart disease.

   _____

   _____

   _____

2. Explain the acronym "ABC" utilized for CPR, and write a brief summary for each component.

   _____

   _____

   _____

   _____

3. a. Define hypovolemic shock. _____

   b. List a few common causes. _____

   c. What is the standard treatment? _____

4. A cat presents with the following clinical signs: polyuria, polydipsia, polyphagia, weight loss, depression, dehydration, weakness, tachypnea, vomiting, and sweet acetone odor to the breath.

   a. What is the most probable diagnosis? _____

   b. What are the primary treatment goals? _____

5. What are the classic laboratory findings in a patient with Addison's disease (hypoadrenalcorticism)?

   _____

   _____

   _____

   _____

1.

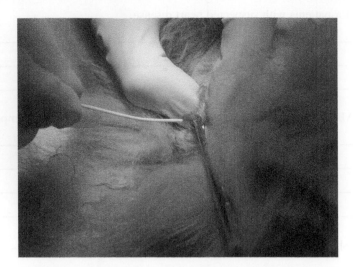

1. Why is this type of catheter being used? _____

2. What is the reason for using the hemostats in this procedure? _____

3. Once the obstruction has been removed, why is it often necessary to replace this type of catheter with a different type? _____

4. For indwelling urinary catheters, is it necessary to have a collection system? _____

2.

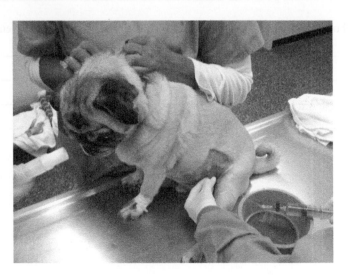

1. What procedure is being performed in the photo above? _____

2. Why is oxygen being administered to this patient? _____

3. What is the correct medical term for this type of fluid build-up? _____

4. Name a common disease that can cause this type of abdominal effusion. _____

3.

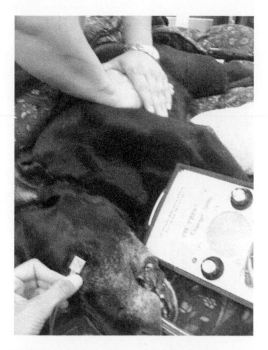

What is the purpose of the Doppler as it is being used in the photo above? _____

4.

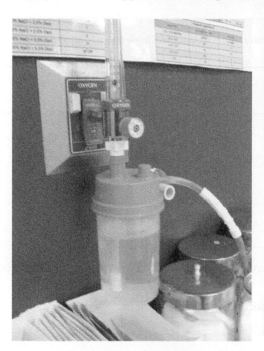 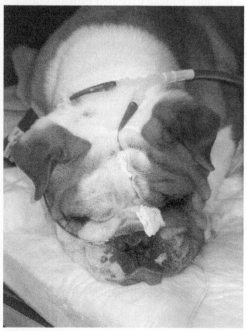

1. Why is the apparatus on the left necessary with nasal oxygen insufflation? _____

2. What is the advantage of using two nasal oxygen lines? _____

3. What are some options to increase oxygen flow in this patient if nasal oxygen is not working?

_____

_____

4. Are there any contraindications to nasal oxygen?

_____

_____

5.

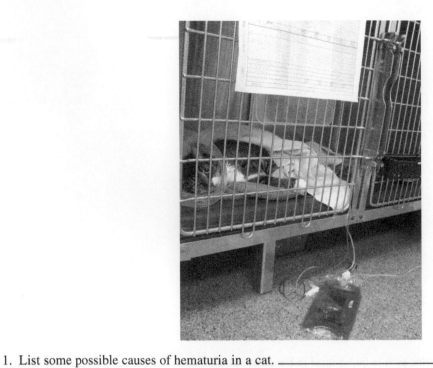

1. List some possible causes of hematuria in a cat. _____

2. What is the approximate expected urinary output? _____

3. If the urinary output is decreased, what can the technician do to trouble shoot the situation?

_____

FILL IN THE BLANK

Choose from words listed below.

- Dyspnea
- Sterile
- Nebulization
- ACTH stimulation
- Thoracocentesis
- Hyperkalemia
- Hypoxemia
- Fluid
- Brainstem
- Pulse oximetry

1. Indications for oxygen administration include _____, or a PaO_2 <60 mm Hg.

2. _____ is a simple, useful procedure for collection of pleural fluid to obtain samples for diagnostic evaluation or for alleviation of respiratory distress.

3. _____ technique is indicated to prevent nosocomial infection in all invasive procedures.

4. Clinical signs of hypoxia include cyanosis, tachycardia, and _____.

5. Diagnosis of hypoadrenalcorticism is typically by an _____ test.

6. _____ is a common sequela to urinary obstruction.

7. _____ promotes bronchial drainage by liquefying thick respiratory secretions.

8. Acute changes in weight are usually a result of _____ changes as opposed to muscle mass.

9. Irregular breathing patterns may indicate _____ disease or high cervical trauma.

10. _____ is a noninvasive technique that continuously measures arterial oxygen saturation in the blood.

Circle all that could apply in the following.

1. Tachycardia

   - hypovolemia
   - heart disease in the cat
   - fever
   - excitement
   - high vagal tone
   - exercise
   - heart disease in the dog
   - pain

2. Bradycardia

   - high vagal tone,
   - severe electrolyte disturbances
   - hypovolemia
   - heart disease in the cat
   - pain
   - atrioventricular conduction blocks

3. Pleural effusion

   - increased CVP
   - decreased CVP
   - hyperactivity
   - dull mentation
   - normal respiratory rate
   - increased lung sounds
   - decreased lung sounds
   - muffled heart sounds
   - poor pulse quality
   - anisocoria
   - SaO_2 >95%

4. Poor perfusion

   - altered mental state
   - abnormal temperature
   - abnormal heart rate
   - increased urinary output
   - bounding pulses
   - weak pulses
   - tachypnea
   - irregular breathing pattern
   - pale gray mucous membranes
   - brick-red mucous membranes
   - prolonged capillary refill time
   - hyperactivity
   - cool extremities

5. Chronic heart disease

   - injected, pale, or cyanotic mucous membranes
   - obesity
   - dull lung sounds on auscultation
   - crackles
   - wheezes
   - poor jugular filling
   - head tilt
   - jugular venous distension
   - anisocoria,
   - labored breathing
   - hyperactivity
   - poor pulse quality
   - pulse deficits
   - abnormal heart rate
   - ascites
   - hyperthermia
   - coughing

Identify the term described and then find the words in the Word Search.

1. Hypoadrenocorticism _____

2. Listening for abnormal heart or lung sounds _____

3. Increased BUN _____

4. Ascites _____

5. Method of removing secretions from lower airway _____

6. Difficult birthing process _____

7. Decreased intravascular volume _____

8. Poor oxygenation _____

9. Infection not existing at time of admission _____

10. Decreased urine production _____

11. Abnormal neurologic posture _____

12. Pus in uterus _____

13. Arterial clot _____

```
P N L N R R B C Y L G Y Q P F C K R Y Y T M
K D N F L Q D F R T N Z F Q L J P C H J Y D
F R J G C W H Y P O V O L E M I C S H O C K
J Y M P Z C W Z S L F H K Z V L K M M P N N
H T T D Z Y E O A M Q M F M F N R D Q H S N
Y C P D D G C R R D Y S T O C I A Y T T U L
R W L N A O T Z L W W Y T M D N K C N K N X
X H K P M E G F N F R Y N A N T G P C K O M
K G U I M X C N Q L T X R I H X N B R T G
T O A O P H P A G N L W N M R T R W V H O T
C L Y D L M Y J D Z D H G E T R C D N Q H N
N P L J T N M F K D F F H T A D B C Q H X
L D W N Y T G M G M I T F O R I F R Z Y S Q
Y N M J G T D F L X L S X Z R L R C T P I P
T L T Q H H P L D J T K O A V L X U N O P V
L M V Z L L L M B Q Z R M N R K J N G X O M
D R V R G N W L X V L Z R L I W G D X I C L
N O I T A T L U C S U A T L N A Q R R A L F
D K R X P T V V L L F Y H K X X N G M N G O
E R U L I A F T R A E H E V I T S E G N O C
W B B P B M K S A D D L E T H R O M B U S H
J T M L R R T J J M K W B G Q W Q N J M T Y
```

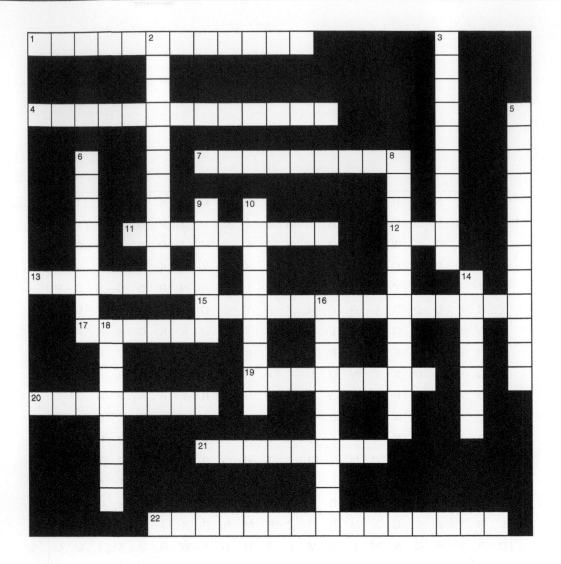

Chapter **17** **Emergency and Critical Care**

Copyright © 2011 by Mosby, Inc., an affiliate of Elsevier Inc.

Across

1 A state of a severe hyperextension and spasticity wherein a patient's head, neck, and spinal column enter into a complete "arching" position. (12)

4 A noninvasive technique that continuously measures arterial oxygen saturation in the blood. (2 words) (13)

7 Deficient oxygenation of blood. (9)

11 The type of care directed toward the assessment, treatment, and stabilization of a patient with an urgent medical problem. (9)

12 The acronym for the cessation of functional ventilation and effective circulation. (3)

13 An abnormal or difficult labor. (8)

15 Hypoadrenocorticism is a deficiency in the production of mineralocorticoid and/or _____ steroid hormones. (14)

17 A/an _____ thrombus is an embolus that breaks loose and occludes one or more branches of the aorta at the aortic trifurcation. (6)

19 Decreased urine production. (8)

20 The type of care that involves intensive monitoring and treatment of an unstable patient with a life-threatening or potentially life-threatening illness or injury. (8)

21 An infection in the uterus. (8)

22 An aortic _____ is an aggregation of platelets and fibrin that acutely migrates and lodges at a distant site in the circulatory system. (15)

Down

2 The shock condition that arises due to decreased intravascular volume. (11)

3 A hospital-acquired infection. (10)

5 Diabetic ketoacidosis is a potentially life-threatening complication in patients with diabetes mellitus, wherein the body switches to burning fatty acids and produces harmful _____ _____. (2 words) (12)

6 A blue coloration of the skin and mucous membranes due to the presence of deoxygenated hemoglobin. (8)

8 Using a stethoscope to evaluate heart and/or lung sounds. (12)

9 Prioritizing treatment based on medical need. (6)

10 Blood flow across all tissues in a body. (9)

14 A technique used in conjunction with nebulization to promote removal of respiratory secretions. (7)

16 The type of heart failure that results from increased pulmonary or systemic venous capillary pressure, leading to fluid leakage and subsequent pulmonary edema or effusion. (10)

18 An increase in waste products in the blood. (8)

18 Dentistry

LEARNING OBJECTIVES

After reviewing the following chapter, the reader will be able to:
- Describe the normal anatomy of a tooth and the surrounding structures
- List the dental formulas of companion animals
- List and describe the instruments and equipment used during a routine dental prophylaxis
- List and discuss the steps involved with a dental prophylaxis
- Differentiate between the most common charting systems
- Describe procedures used in basic dental radiology
- Discuss common dental care home care products

TRUE OR FALSE

1. _____ Pets that receive good-quality cleanings and home care stay healthier.

2. _____ Owners do not need to play an active role to keep their pets healthy.

3. _____ To help you quickly identify and record findings in the oral cavity, it is advisable to laminate a reference chart.

4. _____ It is best to evaluate a patient's bite before the patient is intubated.

5. _____ Scaling the calculus off the surface of the tooth leaves the tooth surface smooth.

6. _____ Enamel can regenerate.

7. _____ Cementum can regenerate.

8. _____ A baby tooth is also known as a primary tooth.

9. _____ A baby tooth is also known as a permanent tooth.

10. _____ An adult tooth is known as a deciduous tooth.

11. _____ If extracted improperly, deciduous canines can deflect into an abnormal position.

12. _____ Because the permanent teeth have not developed yet, there are no risks to extracting a deciduous canine.

13. _____ There are no deciduous molars in the kitten or puppy.

14. _____ All stages of periodontal disease are reversible.

15. _____ Good quality, thorough dentals can be performed on a patient that is awake.

16. _____ Quadrants 1 and 5 correspond to the right maxilla.

17. _____ Quadrants 2 and 6 correspond to the left mandible.

18. _____ Quadrants 4 and 7 correspond to the left mandible

19. _____ Quadrants 3 and 7 correspond to the left mandible.

20. _____ It is best to learn and use both the Alphanumeric and Triadan systems for charting the oral cavity.

1. Match the stage of periodontal disease with its description.

1. _____ Stage 1   A. pocket depth of 9mm (dog)/1.5mm (cat) and 50% attachment loss

2. _____ Stage 2   B. pocket depth >9mm (dog)/1.5mm (cat) and >50% attachment loss

C. inflammation, mild gingivitis, no attachment loss

3. _____ Stage 3   D. pocket depth of 5mm (dog)/1mm (cat), 25% attachment loss

4. _____ Stage 4

2. Match the correct number of teeth to the correct tooth type and species.

1. _____ Feline deciduous   A. 30

2. _____ Feline permanent   B. 26

C. 28

3. _____ Canine deciduous   D. 42

4. _____ Canine permanent

3. Match the skull type with the description.

1. _____ Mesaticephalic   A. long, narrow face

2. _____ Brachycephalic   B. short, wide face

C. average, proportional face

3. _____ Dolichocephalic

4. Match the skull type with a common breed example.

1. _____ Mesaticephalic   A. Labrador

2. _____ Brachycephalic   B. Collie

C. Boxer

3. _____ Dolichocephalic

5. Match the following dental hand instrument to the correct purpose.

1. _____ Sickle scaler   A. used to determine depth of sulcus or pocket

2. _____ Probe   B. used to detect softened areas in enamel

C. used to scale calculus off the crown of the tooth

3. _____ Explorer   D. used to remove calculus subgingivally

4. _____ Curette

6. Match the adult tooth quadrants with their corresponding number.

1. _____ 1   A. Left mandible

2. _____ 2   B. Right mandible

C. Left maxilla

3. _____ 3   D. Right maxilla

4. _____ 4

7. Match the primary tooth quadrants with their corresponding number.

1. _____ 5   A. Left mandible

2. _____ 6   B. Right mandible

C. Left maxilla

3. _____ 7   D. Right maxilla

4. _____ 8

8. Match the triadan tooth number with the correct tooth.

1. _____ 01   A. Canine
2. _____ 06   B. Second premolar
                 C. First incisor
3. _____ 10   D. Second molar
4. _____ 04

9. Match the triadan tooth number with the correct tooth.

1. _____ 03   A. First premolar
2. _____ 07   B. Third premolar
                 C. Third incisor
3. _____ 09   D. First molar
4. _____ 05

10. Match the triadan tooth number with the correct tooth.

1. _____ 11   A. Fourth premolar
2. _____ 02   B. Third molar
                 C. Canine
3. _____ 08   D. Second incisor
4. _____ 04

SHORT ANSWER AND FILL IN BLANKS

1. The oral cavity consists of the teeth, face, lips, gingiva, mucosa, _____, _____ and _____.

2. The primary functional structure(s) of the oral cavity is (are) the _____.

3. The visible portion of a tooth is known as the _____.

4. The submerged portion of the tooth is known as the _____.

5. CEJ is an abbreviation for _____.

6. Enamel is comprised of _____ crystals.

7. The pulp cavity is surrounded by the _____.

8. Blood vessels, nerves, and connective tissues can be found in the _____.

9. The apical delta or delta foramina is found in the _____ area of the tooth.

10. The point where multiple roots connect to the neck of the tooth is known as a/an _____.

11. The three factors that can influence the sequence in which the permanent teeth can erupt are _____, _____ and _____.

12. _____ maintains the stability of the teeth in the oral cavity.

13. The _____ stabilizes the tooth within the socket and absorbs the forces generated by chewing.

14. The space between the tooth and the free gingiva is termed the _____.

15. The normal sulcus depth for a dog is _____.

16. The normal sulcus depth for a cat is _____.

17. Plaque is a soft mixture of bacteria and _____ that adhere to the surface of the tooth.

18. The most commonly used scaling unit is a/an _____ scaler.

19. Ultrasonic scalers produce _____.

20. _____ is used to keep the ultrasonic scaler cool.

21. Prior to administering anesthesia to a patient, the patient should be _____.

22. A dental pack should include _____, _____, _____, _____, tartar removal forceps, and an ultrasonic scaling tip.

23. PPE is an abbreviation for _____ _____ _____.

24. The PPE that a technician should use while performing a dental cleaning includes _____, _____ or _____, and a _____.

25. Calculus contains _____, which can be aerosolized.

26. The process by which the teeth are cleaned is referred to as _____.

27. Bacteria and mineral build-up can cause gingivitis and _____ of the tooth and bone.

28. A prophylaxis is performed in a _____ approach to avoid missing any portion of the dental cleaning.

29. Subgingival scaling is considered _____ in some states and must be performed by the veterinarian.

30. The purpose of subgingival curettage is to remove _____, _____, _____, and _____ from below the gum line.

31. After a subgingival cleaning, the mouth is rinsed with _____ or _____.

32. _____ is used to highlight plaque in a bright pink color.

33. It is best to _____ before stains, sealants, or polish has been applied to the teeth.

34. In some states, technicians are allowed to extract _____ and _____.

35. Grooves on the surface of the tooth increase the _____ of the tooth.

36. The 10 steps to a dental prophylaxis are: 1) examine, 2) ultrasonic scaling, 3) _____, 4) subgingival curette, 5) disclosing liquid & flush, 6) _____/explore, 7) radiographs, 8) _____, 9) _____, 10) sealants.

37. Throughout the process of the prophylaxis, the mouth is continuously evaluated for _____.

38. The oral cavity is evaluated _____, during, and _____ the prophylaxis.

39. Two commonly used charting systems are _____ and _____.

40. The triadan system is based on a _____ -digit number that corresponds with each tooth.

41. The first digits of the triadan system pertaining to the adult mouth are _____, _____, _____, and _____.

42. The first digits of the triadan system pertaining to the primary teeth are _____, _____, _____, and _____.

43. The first digit of the _____ system refers to the quadrant of the mouth.

44. The alphanumeric charting system is made up of abbreviations that _____ correspond to the tooth's name.

45. The abbreviation for an incisor is _____.

46. The abbreviation for a molar is _____.

47. The abbreviation *C* in the alphanumeric system stands for _____.

48. The abbreviation *PM* in the alphanumeric system stands for _____.

49. To identify and differentiate between each premolar, a _____ is placed next to the abbreviation PM.

50. To identify and differentiate between each incisor, a number is placed next to the abbreviation of _____.

51. Your medical record states the first incisor on the right maxilla was extracted. Using the triadan system, this is tooth # _____, and in the alphanumeric system it is identified as tooth _____.

52. Your medical record states the second molar on the left mandible was extracted. Using the triadan system, this is tooth # _____, and in the alphanumeric system it is identified as tooth _____.

53. Your medical record states the fourth premolar on the left maxilla was extracted. Using the triadan system, this is tooth # _____, and in the alphanumeric system it is identified as tooth _____.

54. Your medical record states the canine on the right mandible was extracted. Using the triadan system, this is tooth # _____, and in the alphanumeric system it is identified as tooth _____.

COMPLETE THE CHART

Dimple placement in the mouth	
View in mouth	**Dimple Placement**
Right maxilla	_____
Left maxilla	_____
If film is parallel to canines	_____
Left mandible	_____
Right mandible	_____
If film is parallel to canines	_____

SHORT ANSWER

Describe the characteristics of each stage of periodontal disease.

1. Stage 1

_____

_____

_____

_____

_____

2. Stage 2

_____

_____

_____

_____

_____

3. Stage 3

_____

_____

_____

_____

_____

4. Stage 4

_____

_____

_____

_____

_____

PHOTO QUIZ _____

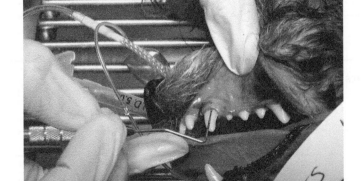

1. Which step of the prophylaxis is this technician performing?

_____

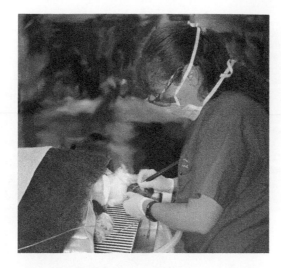

2. List the personal protective equipment that this technician is wearing.

_____

_____

_____

_____

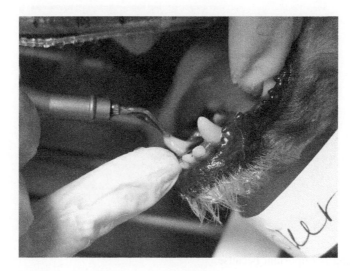

3. What type of scaler is this technician using?

_____

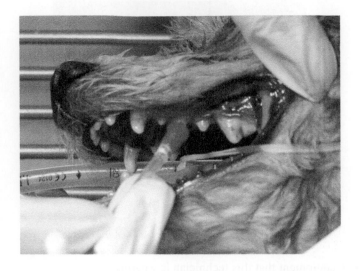

4. What product is being used on this patient?

_____

_____

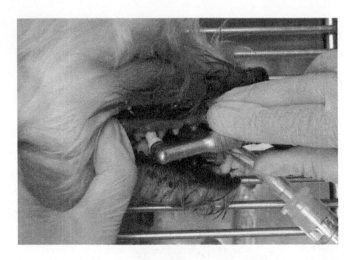

5. Polishing teeth after scaling is important because:

_____

_____

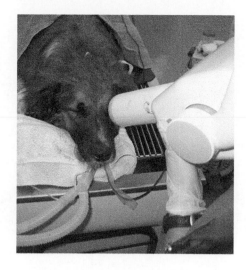

6. Which tooth/teeth is/are being radiographed?

_____

_____

_____

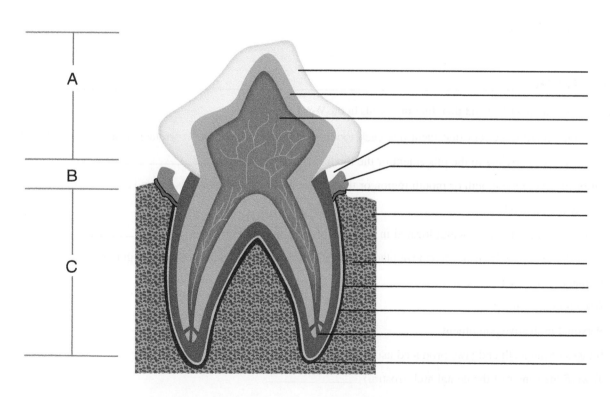

7. Label this figure.

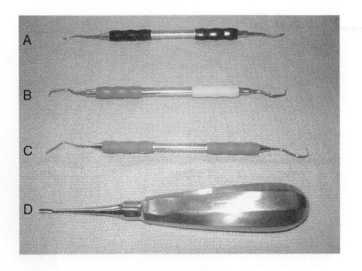

8. Label the instruments pictured.

    a. _____

    b. _____

    c. _____

    d. _____

WORD SEARCH

Identify the term described and then find the words in the Word Search.

1. A dental charting system that identifies each tooth with letters that directly correlate with the type of tooth and numbers that correlate to the placement of the tooth in the dental arcade _____

2. Of or involving the mouth or mouth region or the surface on which the mouth is located _____

3. Below the gingival _____

4. A tooth for cutting or gnawing; located in the front of the mouth in both jaws _____

5. An instrument used by hand to remove plaque and calculus from tooth surfaces above the gum line _____

6. Primary, or first set of, teeth _____

7. A scaling instrument _____

8. Personal protective equipment _____

9. Images of the teeth and jaws produced using x-rays _____

10. Toward the center of the dental arch (rostral) _____

11. The substance that cover the crown of the tooth. It is a substance in the body (96% inorganic) and is made of hydroxyapatite crystals _____

12. The lower jaw or arcade of teeth _____

13. Inflammation of the gingival _____

14. The place where something divides into two branches _____

15. A misalignment of teeth and/or incorrect relation between the teeth of the two dental arches _____

16. Of, pertaining to, or caused by resorption _____

17. The hardened, or calcified, plaque _____

18. The upper jaw or arcade of teeth _____

19. Space between the tooth and the free gingival _____

20. The unexposed, or submerged, portion of the tooth below the gingival tissue _____

21. The process by which the teeth are cleaned to prevent disease _____

22. A dental charting system that identifies each tooth with a three-digit number that corresponds to each tooth _____

23. Surgical removal of a tooth _____

24. The exposed, or visible, portion of the tooth above the gingival tissue _____

25. The inflammation and infection of the gums, ligaments, bone, and other tissues surrounding the teeth _____

26. The broad back teeth, used for grinding food _____

```
A  L  P  H  A  N  U  M  E  R  I  C  I  S  U  B  O  P  O
O  M  E  W  E  R  O  E  R  T  Y  U  E  A  L  P  M  L  C
O  O  R  A  L  A  D  S  U  B  G  I  N  G  I  V  A  L  C
I  F  I  B  N  C  O  I  G  H  I  O  A  O  F  K  N  A  O
T  O  O  C  A  L  N  A  K  A  N  C  M  W  O  Y  D  X  D
I  R  D  N  M  A  T  L  J  X  G  C  E  N  R  T  I  I  O
S  F  O  G  B  S  D  F  G  I  I  I  L  H  A  N  B  S  N
D  I  N  C  I  S  O  R  L  S  V  T  X  I  L  L  L  J  T
Z  P  T  O  F  C  R  Z  M  E  I  I  O  D  T  R  E  G  F
R  R  A  W  U  I  E  O  A  R  T  S  S  C  A  L  E  R  O
E  O  L  N  R  S  L  O  L  T  I  E  U  S  O  R  U  O  R
S  P  D  E  C  I  D  U  O  U  S  A  L  H  P  H  J  O  M
O  H  I  C  A  C  A  L  C  F  I  S  C  U  R  E  T  T  E
R  J  S  U  T  S  O  R  C  J  K  E  U  Y  O  S  R  E  X
P  P  E  R  I  Z  C  B  L  V  K  U  S  T  P  I  I  A  T
T  K  A  R  O  D  R  J  U  E  U  I  I  O  H  T  A  S  R
I  L  S  E  N  F  O  H  S  X  J  T  H  K  Y  I  D  E  A
V  P  E  A  N  G  W  G  I  T  M  A  X  I  L  L  A  I  C
E  X  I  L  L  H  N  D  O  R  O  O  R  W  A  T  N  T  T
S  U  B  S  O  R  J  S  N  A  L  C  A  D  X  Y  H  I  I
S  U  L  U  C  L  A  C  X  C  A  C  C  G  I  I  F  S  O
R  A  D  V  R  A  D  I  O  G  R  A  P  H  S  A  L  P  N
```

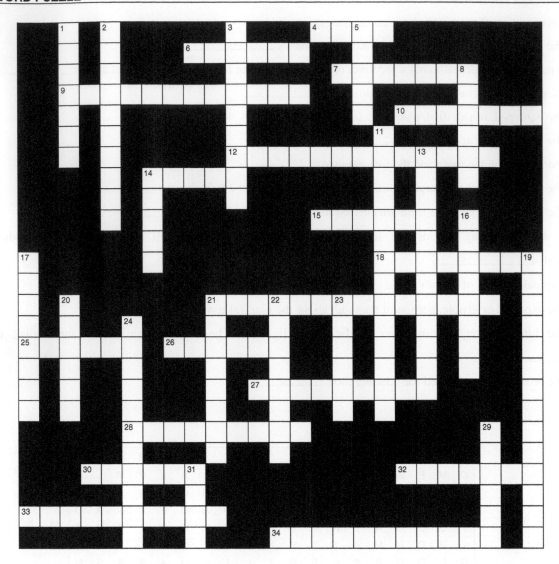

Across

4 A row of teeth. (4)

6 The layer beneath the enamel and cementum of a tooth. (6)

7 In veterinary dentistry this direction is toward the center of the dental arch. (7)

9 A dental charting system that identifies each tooth with a letter that directly correlates with the type of tooth and a number that correlates to the placement of the tooth in the dental arcade. (12)

10 This condition is caused by the mandible and maxilla being different lengths on the right and left sides. (2 words) (7)

12 The surface between two teeth. (13)

14 Permanent teeth are also referred to as _____ or secondary teeth. (5)

15 The tooth surface toward the cheek. (6)

18 The substance that covers the root of a tooth. (8)

21 Having a short, wide muzzle. (14)

25 A soft mixture of bacteria and carbohydrates that adheres to a tooth. (6)

26 In veterinary dentistry this direction is away from the center of the dental arch. (6)

27 The junction where multiple roots join the neck of the tooth. (9)

28 The _____ teeth are the primary or first set of teeth. (9)

30 Maxillary prognathism results from the maxillary arcade being _____ than the mandibular arcade. (6)

32 The upper jaw or arcade of teeth. (7)

33 _____ _____ canines are identified when the angle of the canine growth is directed inward from a normal occlusal. (2 words) (10)

34 Cleaning teeth to prevent disease. (11)

Down

1 A dental charting system that identifies each tooth with a three-digit number that corresponds to that tooth. (7)

2 The delta foramina (apical delta) is the entry point for the nerves and blood vessels into the _____ _____. (2 words) (10)

3 Another term for maxillary brachygnathism. (9)

5 The exposed or visible portion of a tooth above the gingival tissue. (5)

8 The tooth surface toward the lips. (6)

11 Having a long, narrow muzzle. (14)

13 Gingivitis refers to _____ of the gingiva. (12)

14 The bisecting _____ technique is a radiographic technique in which the film is placed as close to the intended tooth as possible and the cone is directed midway between the angle of the tooth and the film. (5)

16 The lower jaw or arcade of teeth. (8)

17 Interdigitations of connective tissue that provide a firm attachment to the periosteum of the alveolar bone. (2 words) (8)

19 Having a medium length and width muzzle. (14)

20 The substance that covers the crown of the tooth. (6)

21 _____ _____ canines are identified when the angle of the canine growth is directed outward from a normal occlusal. (2 words) (8)

22 The hardened or calcified plaque on teeth. (8)

23 With an anterior crossbite the maxillary incisors are _____ to the mandibular incisors. (6)

24 The _____ ligament holds the tooth in the alveolar bone. (11)

29 The gingival _____ is the space between the free gingiva and the enamel of the tooth. (6)

31 The unexposed portion of a tooth below the gingival tissue. (4)

19 Physical Therapy, Rehabilitation, and Complementary Medicine

After reviewing this chapter, the reader will be able to:
- Differentiate between vibrational hands-on and manipulation hands-on therapies
- Describe the benefits of physical therapy and rehabilitation
- Discuss appropriate uses for thermal therapy
- Describe the differences in massage types and variations of applications
- Describe the concepts of passive range of motion therapy and active exercise for rehabilitation
- Define Allopathic medicine
- Differentiate between alternative and complementary therapies
- Discuss similarities in various cultural philosophies of energy and healing modalities
- List and describe commonly used veterinary complementary therapies
- Describe the concepts of traditional Chinese medicine
- List and describe the theories, techniques, and uses of acupuncture
- Describe contraindications and adverse reactions to acupuncture
- Describe the cultural origins and uses of herbal therapy and define terms used in herbal therapy
- Discuss concepts of aromatherapy and list therapeutic uses of aromatherapy in veterinary medicine
- Discuss flower essences history, theories and uses

SHORT ANSWER OR FILL IN THE BLANK

1. CAVM is also known as IVM because it combines _____ therapies with conventional veterinary therapies such as _____.

2. Three adverse reactions to acupuncture include:

   _____

   _____

   _____

3. TCM is based on the philosophy that _____ _____ cause illness.

4. Western practitioners explain acupuncture's efficacy as stimulating nerves and triggering the release of _____ and _____, which aid in healing.

5. Four topical applications of aromatherapy include:

   _____

   _____

   _____

6. The aromatic properties of essential oils affect the _____ portion of the brain, which governs _____ and _____.

7. Acupuncture is contraindicated in cases of:

_____

_____

_____

8. When scenting a room, essential oils can be used in:

_____

_____

_____

9. Examples of carrier oils suitable for use with animals are:

_____

_____

_____

10. In Traditional Chinese Medicine (TCM), functional properties of herbs include:

_____

_____

_____

_____

_____

11. Combinations of herbs used in TCM are known as _____.

12. Ayurveda is a combination of _____, _____ and _____.

13. Should homeopathic remedies be combined? Why or why not?

_____

_____

_____

_____

_____

14. Homeopathy is contraindicated in conjunction with:

_____

_____

15. Homeopathy is compatible with:

_____

_____

16. Dr. Bach recognized that flowers have qualities that can:

_____

_____

17. Flower essence potency can be increased by:

_____

_____

18. Give two examples of hands-on vibrational therapies.

_____

_____

19. Give three examples of hands-on manipulation therapies.

_____

_____

_____

20. Name three types of rehabilitation therapies commonly used in veterinary medicine.

_____

_____

_____

21. Heat therapy is contraindicated for acute injuries because it _____ _____.

22. Cold therapy treatments should not last longer than _____ minutes due to increase in _____.

23. Hot pack temperatures should range from _____ to _____ °F.

24. How often should the skin be checked when using heat therapy?

_____

_____

_____

25. List four benefits of heat therapy.

1. _____

2. _____

3. _____

4. _____

26. In combination thermal therapy, _____ should be applied before exercise and _____ should be applied after exercise.

27. Tellington TTouch is used as behavior modification based on the theory that:

_____

_____

_____

28. Hydrotherapy should start _____ days postsurgery.

29. Hydrotherapy contraindications include:

_____

_____

_____

30. Passive hydrotherapy water temperature should range from _____ to _____°F.

31. Active hydrotherapy water temperature should range from _____ to _____°F.

32. Spinal adjustments are usually _____ _____ thrusts to an affected _____.

33. Name a calming essential oil that is useful for separation anxiety.

_____

_____

_____

34. List three antibacterial essential oils.

_____

_____

_____

35. Name the five flower essences found in the Bach Flower Rescue Remedy®.

_____

_____

_____

_____

36. Name the flower essence that would be beneficial for wild, feral, or trapped animals.

_____

37. Which flower essence may be beneficial for cats that spray to mark their territory?

_____

38. Class IV therapy lasers are capable of outputs from _____ to _____ watts.

39. List some conditions that can be treated using therapeutic lasers.

_____

_____

40. The primary safety concern when using therapeutic lasers is protection of the _____ of all individuals nearby during therapy.

TRUE OR FALSE

If the statement is false, rewrite the statement to make it true.

1. _____ Complementary and alternative therapies are also referred to as allopathic therapies.

2. _____ All complementary therapy modalities covered in this chapter can be practiced by veterinary technicians.

3. _____ In TCM, meridians of energy flow along acupoints known as qi points.

4. _____ Yin and yang complement each other and should be balanced.

5. _____ Cats tend to react to acupuncture needle placement more than dogs.

6. _____ Acupuncture is considered to be a surgical procedure. Therefore veterinary technicians cannot practice acupuncture.

7. _____ Essential oils are nonoily, concentrated, and very aromatic.

8. _____ Hydrosols are more concentrated than essential oils and should be used with caution.

9. _____ It is not necessary to dilute essential oils for topical use in animals.

10. _____ Aromatherapy is not recommended for use in exotics.

11. _____ Herbal therapies assist in the healing process; they are not always considered to be the cure.

12. _____ All herbs are nutritious and contain vitamins and minerals.

13. _____ Modern Western medicine is in part based on plants and herbs.

14. _____ Homeopathic remedies should be continued until the animal is completely healed.

15. _____ Flower essences are compatible with other modalities and are safe to use for animals.

16. _____ Flower essence potency is increased by adding more drops to the dosage.

17. _____ Reiki can be practiced from a distance.

18. _____ Therapeutic benefits of hypothermia (cold therapy) include localized vasodilation.

19. _____ When performing massage, always direct strokes away from the heart.

20. _____ Tellington TTouch uses massage techniques but is not considered to be a realignment method.

DEFINITION

Define the Following Terms:

1. CAVM

   _____

   _____

2. IVM

   _____

   _____

3. AVMA

   _____

   _____

4. TCM

_____

_____

5. IVAS

_____

_____

6. Acupuncture

_____

_____

7. Acupressure

_____

_____

8. Aromatherapy

_____

_____

9. Reflexology

_____

_____

10. Essential oil

_____

_____

11. Hydrosol

_____

_____

12. Herbal therapy

_____

_____

13. Zoopharmacognosy

_____

_____

14. Dosha

_____

_____

15. Compress

_____

_____

16. Succussion

_____

_____

17. Healing crisis

_____

_____

18. Rescue Remedy®

_____

_____

19. Passive exercise

_____

_____

20. Effleurage

_____

_____

21. Petrissage

_____

_____

22. Passive hydrotherapy

_____

_____

23. Subluxation

_____

_____

Chapter **19** **Physical Therapy, Rehabilitation, and Complementary Medicine**

Term for Life Force Energy	Country of Origin	Modality
	China	
Ki		Reiki
Prana	India	

Massage Benefits	Massage Contraindications

MATCHING

Traditional Chinese Medicine (TCM)

1. _____ Qi
2. _____ Meridians
3. _____ Yin
4. _____ Yang
5. _____ Moxibustion
6. _____ Acupuncture
7. _____ Acupressure
8. _____ Sonapuncture

A. Calm, dark, moon
B. Placing of needles into acupoints
C. Use of heat to stimulate acupoints
D. Channels found throughout the body
E. Unyielding, active, sun
F. Use of ultrasound to stimulate acupoints
G. Using fingers to stimulate acupoints
H. Life force energy

Herbal Therapies

1. _____ Single herb remedies
2. _____ Herb combinations
3. _____ An herb known for effectiveness in treatment of a particular condition
4. _____ Herbal infusion
5. _____ Liquid herbal extract preserved with alcohol
6. _____ Wet herbal pack
7. _____ Hot herbal compress

A. Blends
B. Tisane
C. Simples
D. Poultice
E. Fomentation
F. Tincture
G. Specific

Massage

1. _____ Enhances lymph drainage

2. _____ Stretches muscles and tendons

3. _____ Helps loosen superficial scar tissue

4. _____ Helps maintain skin tone

A. Petrissage
B. Stretch pressure massage
C. Effleurage
D. Friction massage

WORD SEARCH

Identify the term described and then find the words in the Word Search.

1. Metabolic body type used in Ayurveda to determine balances and imbalances _____

2. TCM term describing female energy—calm, yielding, stillness, darkness, water, and moon _____

3. Rivers or channels that travel throughout a body connecting and regulating different body parts and organs

_____

4. Use of finger pressure instead of needles on acupoints along body meridians _____

5. Placing of small, sharp, sterile needles into specific points on the body _____

6. Use of water as physical therapy _____

7. Another term used to describe Western medicine _____

8. Practices that deviate from the Western approach _____

9. Therapeutic use of pure essential oils derived from aromatic plants to help balance and heal the mind, body, and

spirit _____

10. Deep massage used on back, flank, and chest; skin is lifted, pulled, and kneaded _____

11. East Indian philosophy of diet, herbs, and exercise used to promote health and vitality _____

12. Hot compress _____

13. Spinal adjustments performed to reverse a variety of nerve, muscle, and motion problems _____

14. Practices used in conjunction with or as complement to Western approach _____

15. No voluntary muscle activity is used during this type of physical therapy _____

16. Use of hand and finger pressure to massage and stimulate pressure points located in the paws _____

17. Cold herbal tea on a cloth _____

18. Wet herbal pack _____

19. Massage technique using palm and fingers in a light and slow motion _____

20. Liquid herbal extracts usually preserved with alcohol or vegetable glycerin _____

21. Therapy that uses specific plant leaves, roots, and/or flowers to assist healing _____

22. A system of healing that uses dilute substances known to cause the same symptoms as the illness

    _____

23. Water left behind after the steam distillation process of aromatherapy _____

24. A tincture that is a natural source combined with alcohol—a term used in homeopathy and flower essences

    _____

25. Chinese term for central life force _____

26. Japanese hands-on energy healing practice that promotes the flow of energy to aid in the healing process

    _____

27. Misalignment of vertebrae causing compensation in posture or movement _____

28. Use of heat or cold to facilitate circulation and pain relief _____

29. Herbal infusion _____

30. TCM term describing male energy—insistent, unyielding, activity, brightness, fire, and sun _____

```
A R O M A T H E R A P Y Z K V Q K T U
F L A F O M E N T A T I O N J G T H A
S H L M E R I D I A N S K Y H E H O Q
Z U Y O H Y D R O T H E R A P Y E M C
E C B D P M K U C X Z G K F Q H R E O
T H C L R A A Y U R V E D A P H M O Y
R I G M U O T L O R E M Q A D Y A P H
E R W C O X S H T C X F L T R O L A E
F O Z Y Y T A O I E O B N A I B S T R
L P Z I K L H T L C R M T C I S L H B
E R T N F C L E I S T N P X I F A Y A
X A I M L U O U R O E E A R R T J N L
O C N M O X C N D M N S V T E P Q M E
L T C P E F F L E U R A G E I S I O O
O I T T I B G L P A S S I V E V S K T
G C U A C U P U N C T U R E E Y E K Z
Y U R I Y M X M W R E I K I U A Q U I
H X E Y O P E T R I S S A G E N W S S
I K A C U P R E S S U R E T P G O E X
```

Chapter **19** **Physical Therapy, Rehabilitation, and Complementary Medicine**

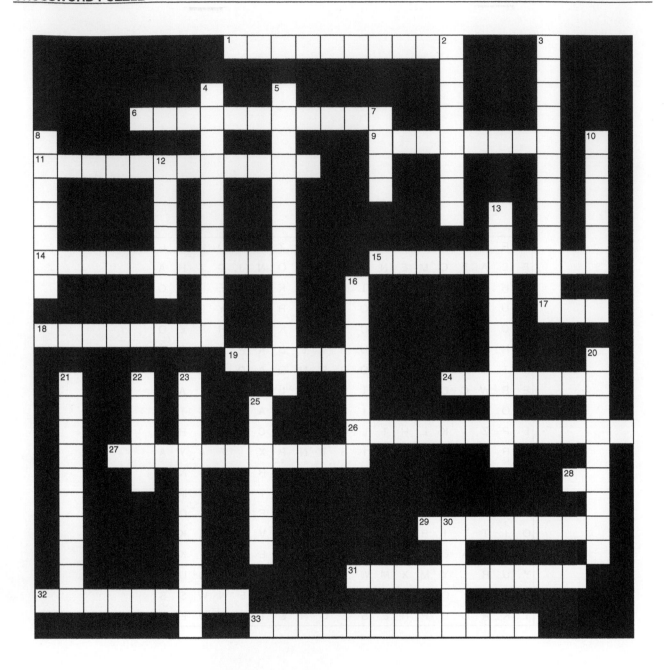

Across

1 Another term used to describe traditional "Western" medicine. (10)

6 The use of hand and finger pressure to massage and stimulate pressure points located in the paws. (11)

9 East Indian philosophy of diet, herbs, and exercise used to promote health and vitality. (8)

11 The use of water as physical therapy. (12)

14 Placing small, sharp, sterile needles into specific points on the body. (11)

15 A massage technique using the palm and fingers in a light slow motion. (10)

17 A traditional Chinese medicine term describing female energy. (3)

18 A liquid herbal extract usually preserved with alcohol or vegetable glycerin. (8)

19 The type of therapy that uses specific plant leaves, roots, and/or flowers to assist healing. (6)

24 During __ physical therapy exercise there is no voluntary muscle activity. (7)

26 Spinal adjustments performed to reverse a variety of nerve, muscle, and motion problems. (12)

27 In veterinary medicine the combination of natural and holistic therapies with conventional veterinary therapies. (11)

28 The Chinese term for central life force. (2)

29 A fast, invigorating, circular massage. (8)

31 A deep massage used on the back, flank, and chest. (10)

32 The water left behind after the steam distillation process of aromatherapy. (9)

33 Misalignment of vertebrae causing compensation in posture or movement. (12)

Down

2 Cold herbal tea poured on a cloth. (8)

3 The therapeutic use of pure essential oils derived from certain plants to help balance and heal the mind, body, and spirit. (12)

4 Therapy practices that deviate from the Western approach to medicine. (11)

5 Therapy practices that are used in conjunction with the Western approach to medicine. (13)

7 A traditional Chinese medicine term describing male energy. (4)

8 A type of therapy that uses heat or cold to facilitate circulation and pain relief. (7)

10 A remedy that consists of a single herb. (6)

12 An herbal infusion. (6)

13 The use of finger pressure instead of needles on acupoints along body channels. (11)

16 A wet herbal pack. (8)

20 Channels that travel throughout a body connecting and regulating different body parts and organs. (9)

21 A system of healing that uses dilute substances known to cause the same symptoms as the illness. (10)

22 A remedy that consists of a combination of herbs. (5)

23 Use of a hot compress. (11)

25 A __ crisis occurs when there is a worsening of symptoms followed by overall improvement. (7)

30 A Japanese hands-on energy healing practice that promotes the flow of energy to aid in the healing process. (5)

Chapter **19** **Physical Therapy, Rehabilitation, and Complementary Medicine**

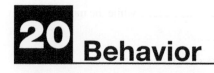

Behavior

LEARNING OBJECTIVES

After reviewing this chapter, the reader will be able to:
- Describe the processes by which behaviors develop
- Differentiate between positive and negative reinforcement and punishment
- List and describe types of aggressive behavior that may be seen in dogs and cats
- Describe the role of veterinary professionals in preventing behavior problems
- List the steps in house training a puppy
- Describe proper litter box care
- List the different options cats look for in scratching posts
- Describe the role of veterinary professionals in managing behavior problems
- List and give examples of various behavior modification techniques
- Describe the procedure for referring clients to professionals for resolution of behavior problems

FILL IN THE BLANK

1. For any behavior to occur, there must be a _____.

2. Some problem behaviors are due to _____ or _____ amounts of neurotransmitters.

3. The study of animal behavior is referred to as _____.

4. _____ conditioning refers to the association of stimuli that occurs at approximately the same time or in roughly the same area as the behavior.

5. _____ conditioning refers to the association of a particular activity with a punishment or reward.

6. The most important time period for behavior development in dogs and cats is from _____ to _____ weeks.

7. Genetics can play a role in behavior problems but also _____ can cause inappropriate behavior.

8. _____ reinforcement refers to any immediate pleasant occurrence that follows a behavior.

9. _____ reinforcement refers to any immediate unpleasant occurrence used to create a desired behavior.

10. _____ is used to remove or decrease a behavior.

11. Positive punishment involves adding an _____ occurrence to decrease a behavior.

12. _____ punishment involves removing a desirable occurrence to decrease a behavior.

13. A delay of longer than _____ seconds between the behavior and the subsequent reinforcement significantly decreases the effectiveness of the reinforcement.

14. _____ refers to the attribution of human characteristics and emotions to animals.

15. Eight-week-old puppies cannot hold their bowels for longer than _____ to _____ hours.

16. One of the most important motivations for cats scratching objects with their front claws is _____ marking.

17. The most common complaint from dog owners is aggression toward _____, while the most common complaint from cat owners is aggression toward other _____.

18. The sensitive socialization period in dogs it is from _____ to _____ weeks of age and in cats from _____ to _____ weeks.

19. When assessing a case of behavior problems, medical conditions that may account for the behavioral signs should first be evaluated. This is especially important with _____ and _____.

20. Behavior modification is needed to accompany _____ to increase the chances of a successful resolution of the problem.

21. _____ who meet the established criteria may become board certified by the American College of Veterinary Behavior and are considered behavior specialists.

22. _____ refers to a repetitive action in which a horse grasps a solid object with its incisors and produces a distinct grunting noise.

CIRCLE THE BEST ANSWER

1. Kittens (**do/do not**) (circle one) need to observe the queen eliminating in the litter box in order to know how to use it properly.

2. Studies have found that cats with elimination problems were more likely to have (**scented/unscented**) (circle one) litter as compared to cats without such problems.

3. It is recommended that in multiple cat households there should be one litter box per (**each/every two cat(s)**) (circle one) plus one.

4. The average age of young (**boys/girls**) (circle one) bitten by dogs is 5 to 9 years old.

5. (**Male/Female**) (circle one) dogs are reported to be involved with 70% to 75% of all reported dog bites.

SHORT ANSWER

1. Give an example of positive reinforcement.

_____

_____

_____

2. Give an example of negative punishment.

_____

_____

_____

3. Describe how a person anthropomorphizes a pet's actions.

_____

_____

_____

4. When are the best times to take a puppy or dog out to eliminate?

_____

_____

_____

5. Explain why the owner must go outdoors with the puppy to be successful in reinforcing elimination versus just waiting by the door.

_____

_____

_____

6. Give the general guidelines owners should follow for maintaining a good litter box environment.

1. _____

2. _____

3. _____

4. _____

7. What unexpected behavior may happen if an owner catches a cat in the litter box in order to administer medications?

_____

_____

_____

8. The scratching objects must match the cat's preferences for the following criteria. Give a recommendation or an example for each criterion.

Desirable location

_____

_____

Height

_____

_____

Orientation

_____

_____

Texture

_____

_____

9. List four of the seven agonistic behaviors identified for both dogs and cats.

   1. _____

   2. _____

   3. _____

   4. _____

10. Give three examples of a variety of situations puppies and kittens should be exposed to in order to prevent fearfulness.

   1. _____

   2. _____

   3. _____

11. Describe the best way to make a behaviorist referral to a client.

   _____

   _____

   _____

WORD SEARCH

Identify the term described and then find the terms in the Word Search.

1. A natural or synthetic chemical that may influence the behavior of an animal _____

2. A veterinarian who is board certified in animal behavior by the American College of Veterinary Behaviorists

   _____

3. An internal or external change that exceeds a threshold, causing stimulation of the nervous or endocrine systems

   _____

4. Any act done by an animal; exhibited for a reason and with purpose _____

5. Attributing human characteristics and emotions to animals _____

6. Behavior that is intended to harm another individual _____

7. Behavioral theory based on the principle that the consequences of a behavior will influence its frequency

   _____

8. Behaviors shown in situations of social conflict to diffuse aggressive behavior _____

9. Exposure of a young animal to new experiences, people, animals, and places with the goal of preventing fearful or anxious behavior as adults _____

10. Female cat, intact; mother cat _____

11. Material selected or preferred by an animal for urination and defecation _____

12. Passing of urine or feces _____

13. Rapid learning process that enables a newborn animal to recognize and bond with its caretaker _____

14. Something that decreases the likelihood of a behavior occurring _____

15. Something that increases the likelihood of a behavior occurring _____

16. The study of animal behavior _____

```
E  Z  S  G  M  N  A  N  H  E  U  M  Q  Y  O  B  E  H  A  V  I  O  R  P  T
N  L  D  O  E  J  N  B  U  E  L  S  E  Y  V  J  A  N  Z  H  D  O  W  N  U
O  S  O  C  I  A  L  I  Z  A  T  I  O  N  M  H  S  S  U  P  J  Y  E  O  X
M  R  R  S  S  W  T  Z  U  I  K  H  M  X  N  U  G  Z  N  I  M  M  C  H  C
O  F  A  M  Z  I  K  D  R  L  Y  P  I  I  W  W  T  V  W  K  E  W  M  G  V
R  J  D  Y  U  I  P  N  H  I  J  R  G  R  N  W  C  E  X  C  J  D  M  S  Z
E  G  I  X  S  K  Y  Q  M  G  G  O  L  H  B  A  U  J  R  K  J  W  J  A  D
H  E  N  T  F  P  Q  P  A  P  Z  M  D  V  J  M  T  O  N  A  X  S  S  E  R
P  Z  F  I  B  J  R  G  T  Q  A  O  A  J  H  V  F  I  R  M  E  Z  U  Y  L
C  X  S  D  N  I  F  J  B  Z  H  P  J  K  E  N  D  R  O  T  E  D  X  W  L
C  B  Q  Z  N  O  F  L  G  R  R  O  X  Q  I  S  F  O  A  N  E  S  R  B  F
L  F  K  T  N  I  I  F  R  H  U  R  Y  E  I  Z  C  R  F  H  W  H  H  C  L
Q  E  I  D  G  K  C  T  Y  V  T  H  R  Q  L  G  T  D  M  R  D  R  N  A  F
N  N  T  D  X  O  O  I  I  V  T  T  O  F  J  S  S  Z  O  O  N  A  E  H  U
G  U  R  H  E  W  K  L  T  D  F  N  H  X  B  U  T  R  J  M  Z  G  O  N  X
N  X  Y  O  O  Z  M  O  W  S  N  A  B  U  W  B  I  R  S  M  J  G  J  Y  F
H  R  G  Z  H  L  C  V  T  T  I  O  S  P  U  T  M  J  G  S  W  R  S  J  H
L  C  Y  N  E  X  O  B  X  F  T  N  C  W  U  V  U  F  O  K  Z  E  W  T  U
F  D  A  Y  C  X  U  G  L  J  D  J  O  T  F  V  L  R  H  M  I  S  J  U  E
V  R  X  F  X  Z  G  M  Y  O  V  M  T  G  N  B  U  U  X  Z  B  S  X  G  U
G  O  U  G  A  Z  O  Y  G  T  C  C  S  Y  A  A  S  E  G  J  W  I  W  X  Q
F  Z  Y  R  C  Y  K  L  Z  E  G  U  N  F  R  Z  R  L  W  K  X  O  X  U  H
T  S  I  R  O  I  V  A  H  E  B  Y  R  A  N  I  R  E  T  E  V  N  E  B  E
I  I  H  Y  D  C  P  H  H  T  N  E  M  H  S  I  N  U  P  B  V  E  R  H  Z
Q  V  J  K  K  L  Z  J  H  X  N  C  M  K  C  I  W  A  B  O  N  Q  Y  H  C
```

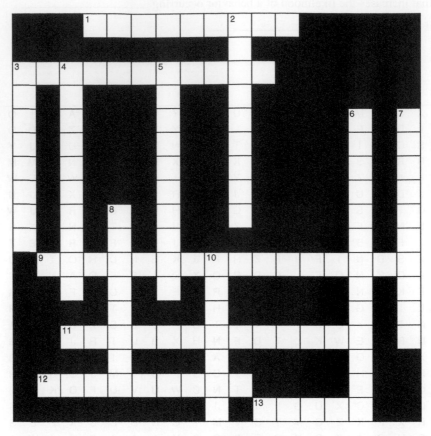

Across

1 Material selected or preferred by an animal for urination or defecation. (9)
3 Passing urine or feces. (11)
9 Attributing human characteristics and emotions to animals. (16)
11 Something that increases the likelihood of a behavior occurring. (13)
12 A natural or synthetic chemical that may influence an animal's behavior. (9)
13 An intact female cat. (5)

Down

2 Behaviors shown in situations of social conflict to diffuse aggressive behavior. (9)
3 The study of animal behavior. (8)
4 Rapid learning process that enables a newborn animal to recognize and bond with its caretaker. (10)
5 Behavior that is intended to harm another individual. (10)
6 Exposure of a young animal to new experiences, people, animals, and places with the goal of preventing fearful or anxious behavior as adults. (13)
7 Something that decreases the likelihood of a behavior occurring. (10)
8 Any act done by an animal; exhibited for a reason and with purpose. (8)
10 __ conditioning is a behavioral theory based on the principle that the consequences of a behavior will influence its frequency. (7)

21 | Physical Restraint

LEARNING OBJECTIVES

After reviewing this chapter, the reader will be able to:
- Describe the psychological principles underlying physical restraint techniques
- Explain and implement the safety precautions taken before and during physical restraint
- Restrain dogs, cats, small mammals, birds, horses, cattle, goats, sheep, and pigs for routine procedures such as physical exams, nursing care, and sample collection
- Give examples of behavior responses of animals to physical restraint
- Correctly identify and use restraint equipment

FILL IN THE BLANK

1. The two most dangerous domestic animal mothers with young at side are _____ and _____.

2. The two animal mothers that will fret and go through fences if separated from their young are _____ and _____.

3. An aggressive dog should be fitted with a _____ before entering the veterinary hospital.

4. To perform a cystocentesis you need to place a dog or cat into _____ recumbency.

5. To restrain a cat you have to use the _____ restraint necessary and do the procedure as _____ as possible.

6. One of the best tools for restraining a cat for venipunctures or injections is a large _____.

7. Never leave a cat on a tabletop inside of a _____ bag.

8. Sometimes you can get a procedure done on a cat by puffing air in its face. This is using a _____ technique.

9. A very angry or wild cat can be sedated inside of a cage by squirting _____ into their mouths.

10. You should not use the fetal or scruff hold on a cat that weighs more than _____ pounds.

11. Because their tails "slip" if grasped, the _____ should never be picked up by the tail.

12. You should always wake _____ before reaching into their cages to handle them.

13. If startled, the _____ can go into an epileptic-like seizure.

14. _____ have such powerful back legs that they can actually break their own backs with a violent kick.

15. Rabbits are never picked up by the _____.

16. In order to "hypnotize" rabbits you tilt their _____ back until they go limp.

17. If a ferret is handled roughly, it can become _____ quickly.

18. Sometimes the only way to get a biting ferret to let go is to _____ it in _____.

19. An instrument used on horses more for discipline than restraint is the _____.

20. Always approach and lead the horse on the near or _____ side.

21. The type of knot used to tie an any animal to an inanimate object is a _____ knot.

22. Cattle with _____ are often very dangerous and have killed many people.

23. The rope halter lead will be on the _____ side of the cow's head.

24. The two pieces of equipment used, but only sparingly, to move cattle are the _____ and the _____ prod.

25. Placing a calf in lateral recumbency is called _____.

26. The best way to lure a herd of goats into a pen is with _____ or _____.

27. Instead of a halter, goats are usually led by a _____.

28. Pigs can become _____ when handled roughly, even on a somewhat cool day.

29. In order to get a blood sample from the jugular vein on a hog, you willl need to use a _____ _____.

30. When drawing blood from a pig, personnel should wear _____ protection.

SHORT ANSWER

1. What is the "Fight or Flight" principle?

   _____

   _____

   _____

2. Describe the body language of dogs if:

   Nervous

   _____

   _____

   _____

   Normal

   _____

   _____

   _____

   Aggressive

   _____

   _____

   _____

3. What hazard is associated with gauntlets and restraint?

   _____

   _____

   _____

4. Explain why you do not want to "puppy talk" when trying to get a dog to behave.

_____

_____

_____

5. Describe removing an aggressive dog from a run.

_____

_____

_____

6. Describe lifting a large dog from the floor to an exam table.

_____

_____

_____

7. What is counterproductive when restraining a cat?

_____

_____

_____

8. What is the body language of a cat that is trying to scare you off?

_____

_____

_____

9. Describe what you can tell from a horse by watching its ears, mouth, head, feet, and tail.

Ears

_____

_____

Mouth

_____

_____

Head

_____

_____

Feet

_____

_____

Tail

_____

_____

10. Describe the various distraction techniques used on horses.

Skin twitch

_____

_____

Eyelid press

_____

_____

Ear hold

_____

_____

Blindfolding

_____

_____

11. Describe how horses and cattle see the world.

_____

_____

_____

_____

12. What animal should be kept away from cows and their calves?

_____

_____

13. Describe getting a ruminant to open its mouth for a balling gun.

_____

_____

14. Why do sheep flock?

_____

_____

15. Describe how to capture a single sheep for treatment.

_____

_____

_____

_____

16. Describe how you would pick up and hold a:

Newborn piglet

_____

_____

50-lb pig

_____

_____

MATCHING

For each of the animals in the left column, identify the elements on the right that can be a source of danger when handling the animal.

You may use an answer more than once, or not at all, and there may be more than one correct answer.

1. _____ Dogs	A. Hooves
2. _____ Cats	B. Toenails
	C. Tusks
3. _____ Horses	D. Head
4. _____ Cattle	E. Flight or running away
	G. Teeth and toenails
5. _____ Sheep	H. Teeth
6. _____ Pigs	I. Hooves and Teeth
7. _____ Rodents	
8. _____ Ferret	
9. _____ Goats	
10. _____ Rabbits	

Select the animal that the statements below *best* describe.

A. Bovine   B. Porcine   C. Eaprine   D. Equine   E. Ovine

1. _____ The males can be very unpredictable, and a novice should not be handling them.

2. _____ When working with the young of this animal, always work within sight of the mother.

3. _____ Agile and vocal and will resist restraint if harsh.

4. _____ Bruising and carcass damage can occur if animal is grabbed by wool.

5. _____ Extremely stubborn, a trait that can be used to hold and move them.

6. _____ Tail-jacking is a useful distraction technique.

7. _____ Feet are extremely dangerous. Either walk up close or out 10 to 12 feet.

8. _____ Able to unlock ropes and gate latches.

9. _____ Never get into a small pen with this mother and her offspring.

10. _____ Has an extremely strong flocking instinct.

Select the instrument that could be used to help restrain an animal for the described procedure.

A. Leash   B. Gauntlet   C. Capture pole   D. Muzzle   E. Restraint bag   F. Towel

G. Twitch   H. Hurdles   I. Halter   J. Chute   K. Stanchion

1. _____ Remove a shy or cowering dog from a cage

2. _____ Tail venipuncture on a beef cow

3. _____ Crazy, angry cat that is hiding under the refrigerator

4. _____ A horse that is throwing its head and needs to be tubed

5. _____ Gentle dairy cow for a jugular venipuncture

6. _____ Scruff an angry Cocker Spaniel (in the back room)

7. _____ Rabbit for an ear vein injection

8. _____ Moving several pigs from one place to another

9. _____ Getting a blood sample from the femoral vein on a cat

10. _____ Moving a horse from one place to another

WORD SEARCH

Identify the term described and then find the words in the Word Search.

1. The main tool of restraint used on horses _____

2. Restraint technique used to relax the hindquarters for rectal palpation and tail bleeding of cows, whereby the base of the tail is lifted straight up _____

3. To take preliminary steps toward an animal _____

4. Danger _____

5. Any act done by an animal; exhibited for a reason and with purpose _____

6. Mechanical restraint device consisting of a metal pip with a cable loop on one end _____

7. Mannerisms, postures, and facial expressions that can be interpreted as unconsciously communicating a person's or an animal's feelings or psychological state _____

8. An increase above the body's temperature caused by such things as drugs, toxins, or external temperatures, such as in heatstroke _____

9. Feline restraint sacks _____

10. Amount of restraint to use on a cat _____

11. Rigid pole with a loop at one end used to move an aggressive or fearful dog to or from a run or cage

    _____

12. Kind of behavior that is intended to harm another individual _____

13. Female animal parents, universally protective _____

14. A restraint device used almost exclusively on beef cattle _____

15. Nylon, leather, or gauze covering placed over an animal's mouth to prevent biting _____

16. Exposure or liability to injury, pain, harm, or loss _____

17. A complex of all the attributes—behavioral, temperamental, emotional and mental—that makes each person and each animal unique _____

18. Protection from harm _____

19. Clinical terms used to describe an animal lying down _____

20. A technique that uses mild pain to draw the attention of an animal away so a procedure can be performed _____

21. The state of being physically constrained _____

22. A dog's expression, exhibited by having ears drawn down and back, showing white around the pupils of the eyes, not making eye contact, and cowering _____

23. Being held by the skin on the back of the neck _____

24. Attack _____

25. Restraint technique whereby the animal is held in position using a leash through a wall anchor or the hinges or the bars on a low cage _____

26. Placing a calf in lateral recumbency _____

27. Restraint apparatus for dairy cows; usually consists of a head gate without sidebars to restrict lateral movement _____

28. Escape _____

29. Small, square restraining pens with a front and back gate _____

30. Heavy leather gloves used to restrain animals _____

31. Meekly obedient or passive _____

```
C W G W J E W L D M O Y K J U N C W S F
F H M N L R U M R R M G F Y R O A V T I
T C U Z I F F Y A N U O T O E I T R E G
K T Z T R B X N Z R H I T J A T B E L H
M U C A E R B H A J L L S H D C A C T T
M I E O S L U U H A D J P D E A G U N D
A F O E G A U G N A L Y D O B R R M U F
A I Z W K K U O U S W N Z W Y T S B A L
E G M B J O S D E F F U R C S S P E G U
B L G R V R A P P R O A C H N I X N L G
K E O R E T H G I L F Z J I U D I C Y S
W S H P E H T A I L J A C K I N G Y T T
G M R A H S T O C K S I N Q N H X A N F
P B K B V C S R C C B C H Y O S N I E L
V B X F M I T I E C C B R G W C A D S A
E D E Y X I O A V P N J S E H R A P N N
M I N I M U M R C E Y N X I T N E M E K
E V I S S I M B U S A H O S G L H S F I
M S H W T U S B Y R L N E E N R A O E N
O K L C G K K O E H S R R M T Z X H D G
```

CROSSWORD PUZZLE

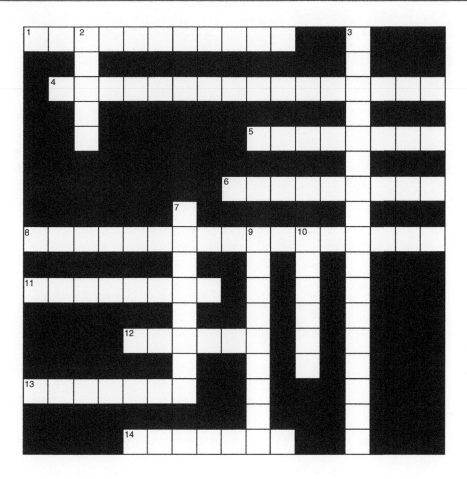

Across

1 A restraint technique that uses mild pain to redirect the attention of an animal so a procedure can be performed. (11)

4 Restraint position whereby the animal is held in place resting on its back. (2 words) (16)

5 A mechanical restraint device consisting of a metal pipe with a cable loop on one end. (2 words) (8)

6 Heavy leather gloves used to restrain animals. (9)

8 Restraint technique whereby the animal is held in position resting on the side of the body. (2 words) (17)

11 Restraint technique whereby the animal is held in position using a leash through a wall anchor or the hinges or bars on a low cage. (8)

12 A chain, rope, or strap that is tightened over a horse's lip as a restraining device. (6)

13 Tail __ is a restraint technique in which the base of the tail is lifted straight up. It used to relax the hindquarters for rectal palpation and tail bleeding of cows. (7)

14 A device used to fasten together the legs of an animal to prevent straying. (7)

Down

2 A small, square restraining pen with a front and back gate. (5)

3 Restraint technique whereby the animal is held in position resting on its breastbone. (2 words) (17)

7 Placing a calf in lateral recumbency. (8)

9 Rigid pole with a loop at one end used to move an aggressive or fearful dog to or from a run or cage. (9)

10 A nylon, leather, or gauze covering placed over an animal's mouth to prevent biting. (6)

Chapter **21** **Physical Restraint**

22 Patient History and Physical Examination

LEARNING OBJECTIVES

After reviewing this chapter, the reader will be able to:
• Discuss the importance of clear communication with the client
• List and describe the components of the patient's history
• Discuss appropriate ways to elicit information from the client
• Describe approaches used for performing the physical examination
• List and describe the components of a physical examination
• Identify methods used to assess patients in emergency situations

FILL IN THE BLANK

1. The interview is most successfully conducted when the technician is _____ but cheerful, friendly, and genuinely concerned about the patient.

2. When conducting a patient history, it is generally more effective to ask _____, _____, and _____ then why.

3. Tapping the body's surface to produce a vibration and sound is called _____.

4. Percussion ventral to the fluid line in the thorax will produce a _____ _____ sound.

5. Percussion dorsal to the fluid line produces a _____ or _____ sound.

6. Listening to sounds produced by the body is termed _____.

7. Relaxation of heart chambers is referred to as _____, and contraction of heart chambers is referred to as _____.

8. The body is normally _____, meaning both sides are complementary or balanced.

9. Vital signs include the _____ rate and effort, _____ rate and rhythm, and indications of _____.

10. A prolonged capillary refill time is more than _____ seconds.

11. Body temperature is maintained by a thermostatic feedback mechanism in the _____.

12. The autonomic nervous system consists of two parts, the _____ _____ and the _____ _____.

13. Cerebral vasoconstriction and brain hypoxia can develop from _____.

14. Body temperature is monitored on animals via the _____.

15. The common passageway for both the digestive and respiratory systems is the _____.

16. The _____ is a flap of cartilage that acts as a "trapdoor" to cover the opening of the larynx during swallowing.

17. Obesity, pericardial effusion, pleural effusion, an intrathoracic mass, or diaphragmatic hernia can muffle _____ sounds.

18. Increased frequency or intensity of intestinal sounds is called _____; decreased frequency or intensity of intestinal sounds is called _____.

19. The term _____ is used to classify patients according to the severity of illness or injury to determine their relative priority for treatment.

20. In an emergency clinic those patients with _____ or _____ issues are treated first.

COMPLETE THE CHART

Animal	Heart Rate (B/M)	Respiration Rate (R/M)	Temperature
Dog			
Cat			
Horse			
Cow			
Sheep			
Pig			
Rabbit			
Hamster			
Guinea Pig			

SHORT ANSWER

1. Why is it important to make sure the gender and age of a patient are correctly recorded on the record?

_____

_____

_____

_____

2. Why is it important to know the geographic origin and prior ownership history on a patient?

_____

_____

_____

_____

3. Why would you ask a client to define a medical term such as stroke to you when taking a history?

_____

_____

_____

_____

4. Describe how to record a patient's history in chronological order.

_____

_____

_____

_____

_____

_____

_____

5. Why is it a good idea to summarize the important parts of the history?

_____

_____

_____

_____

6. What are the four primary techniques employed during a physical exam?

_____

_____

_____

_____

7. What are the six characteristics a technician should note while obtaining the history?

_____

_____

_____

_____

8. Explain how to measure capillary refill and what is considered normal.

_____

_____

_____

_____

9. Using the section on "Systematic Approach to Physical Examination," in the areas below outline what you should be looking for in each.

Head and Neck

_____

_____

_____

_____

Trunk

_____

_____

_____

_____

Limbs

_____

_____

_____

_____

Abdomen

_____

_____

_____

_____

Genitalia and Perineum

_____

_____

_____

_____

10. During an emergency evaluation of the patient, in a primary survey and initial management, life-threatening conditions are addressed in the following order of priority:

_____

_____

_____

_____

11. Describe the following classification system for triage in a multiple animal emergency situation:

Class I

_____

_____

Class II

_____

_____

Class III

_____

_____

Class IV

_____

_____

MATCHING

Match the tactile discrimination with the part of the hand that is best to use when palpating an animal. Draw a line from the description to the part of the hand.

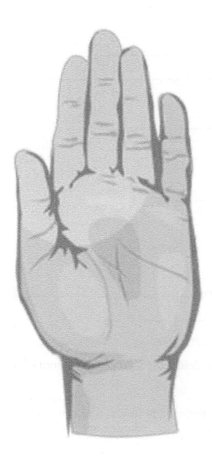

Size and Texture

Vibration

Mobility

Distension

Crepitus

Temperature

Identify the term described and then find the words in the Word Search.

1. The passageway by which air enters and leaves the lungs _____

2. The patient's attentiveness or reaction to its environment _____

3. Critical analysis and evaluation of the status or quality of a particular condition _____

4. To note if the patient appears in normal body condition _____

5. Rhythmically pressing the fist into an area of the abdomen in an attempt to "bump" any large underlying masses or organs _____

6. Noting nonverbal communication, body language, and facial expressions _____

7. The quadrant of the thorax closest to the tail and the back _____

8. The position or carriage of the body _____

9. The quadrant of the thorax closest to the tail and the abdomen _____

10. What the client perceives the patient's problem to be; the primary medical problem _____

11. Pertaining to the neck _____

12. A hollow sound, such as that produced by air-filled lungs _____

13. From the tail _____

14. Acute peripheral circulatory failure _____

15. Relaxation of heart chambers to receive the blood _____

16. Contraction of heart chambers to pump the blood into body tissues and lungs _____

17. A thudlike sound produced by encapsulated tissue, such as liver or spleen _____

18. Pertaining to the chest _____

19. An extremely dull sound produced by very dense tissue, such as muscle or bone _____

20. Also known as the "windpipe," carries air from the larynx to the lungs _____

21. The manner of walking, stepping, or running _____

22. Method used to classify patients according to the severity of illness or injury to determine their relative priority for treatment _____

23. In a clinical examination, the collection of facts about the clinical signs of the patient and its environment (including feeding, vaccination status, and exposure to infection); items in the collection are recorded and arranged in chronological order and in relation to each other _____

24. A musical or drumlike sound produced by an air-filled organ, such as with gastric dilatation-volvulus _____

25. A "booming" sound heard over a gas-filled area, such as an emphysematous lung _____

26. Heard over normal lung parenchyma and produced by movement of air through small bronchi, bronchioles, and alveoli; best heard on inspiration _____

27. Vertebrae between the thoracic vertebrae and the sacrum _____

```
G  S  A  P  Z  P  M  B  N  G  X  O  O  I  S  I  C  R  U  S  D  H  A  T  A
K  G  G  H  D  T  R  O  H  G  B  J  L  D  K  X  K  K  N  Z  M  P  B  N  G
H  R  R  B  T  Q  I  X  I  S  J  X  N  A  N  R  P  F  D  F  A  H  K  I  M
J  A  A  J  W  T  L  K  E  Q  Y  U  L  A  S  R  O  D  O  D  U  A  C  A  T
B  W  T  B  A  G  T  R  K  Z  O  U  U  V  X  W  H  J  N  V  N  V  C  L  F
Y  S  C  T  M  Y  V  U  M  S  Y  R  T  R  D  C  O  V  E  Y  P  I  Y  P  U
L  R  N  J  M  A  H  C  R  M  B  K  M  N  E  L  G  Z  B  C  H  D  F  M  B
M  E  S  P  T  D  L  A  H  Y  P  E  R  R  E  S  O  N  A  N  C  E  A  O  A
M  P  A  I  H  D  L  G  K  L  B  S  M  B  T  M  O  M  M  T  A  A  B  C  M
L  N  O  E  R  U  C  Q  F  H  A  P  Y  B  O  Z  S  N  F  S  Q  P  V  G  L
Y  N  N  F  C  E  E  Y  T  F  Z  J  Q  S  A  I  U  S  A  Z  B  P  N  N  A
S  I  U  I  K  O  R  F  G  X  O  Y  I  B  T  L  R  C  E  N  R  K  I  I  E
A  Y  S  O  A  O  V  D  T  Q  D  R  X  W  L  O  L  A  W  S  C  G  C  T  G
M  E  X  Y  T  U  I  N  U  T  R  I  T  I  O  N  L  O  B  M  S  E  A  N  Y
V  E  O  S  E  A  C  S  S  E  N  L  L  U  D  A  R  E  T  M  U  A  U  E  C
J  J  I  O  S  K  A  A  S  Y  A  W  R  I  A  K  E  G  K  T  U  W  D  S  C
U  H  G  T  C  T  L  L  Q  E  P  O  S  T  U  R  E  A  G  K  E  L  O  E  O
R  L  O  O  I  T  M  B  X  Q  N  B  T  G  A  I  T  I  S  E  R  M  V  R  C
T  L  H  J  C  B  I  B  D  Y  S  T  R  G  V  I  D  R  F  H  H  Q  E  P  W
E  S  G  S  A  P  Q  C  X  C  E  J  A  O  D  M  S  T  W  B  B  G  N  N  A
R  J  W  O  R  D  X  Y  Q  G  V  K  C  L  V  G  M  V  S  K  V  X  T  N  T
D  E  E  Y  O  O  H  Z  G  T  P  Q  H  U  F  U  R  X  O  U  C  U  R  B  E
H  F  P  H  H  C  P  L  G  Z  Y  Q  E  A  Y  W  W  Q  M  I  N  Y  A  Y  W
E  I  Z  E  T  D  X  H  S  L  O  R  A  P  Y  X  I  X  R  W  F  D  L  N  V
A  W  D  Y  B  R  A  T  L  A  T  I  B  U  C  E  E  C  N  A  N  O  S  E  R
```

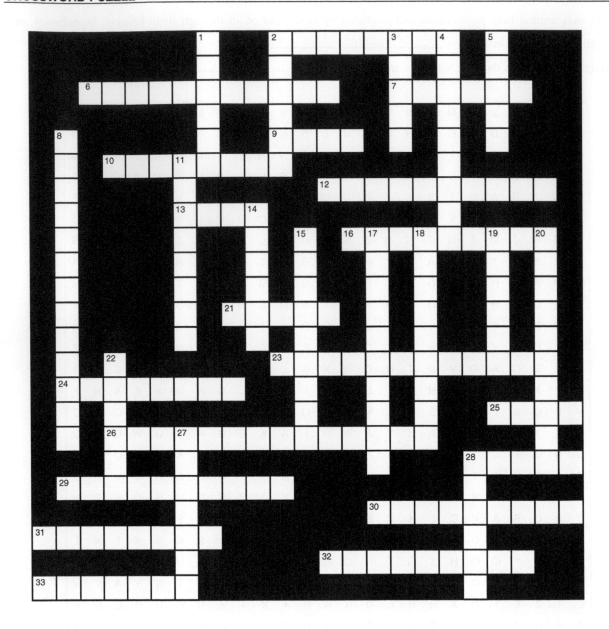

Chapter **22** **Patient History and Physical Examination**

Across

2 The __ vertebrae are located in the chest region and form joints with the dorsal ends of the ribs. (8)

6 A __ diagnosis is made without having all the facts or proof. (11)

7 The fused __ vertebrae are located in the pelvic region. (6)

9 **The manner of walking, stepping, or running. (4)**

10 Conducts impulses received from other neurons toward the nerve cell body. (8)

12 The part of the brain that does not initiate movements but serves to coordinate, adjust, and generally fine-tune movements. (10)

13 Conducts impulses away from a nerve cell body to other neurons or effector organs such a muscle cells. (4)

16 Abnormal and uncontrolled growth of cells. (9)

21 The type of nerve that carries only instructions from the central nervous system out to the body. (5)

23 Rhythmically pressing the fist into an area of the abdomen in an attempt to "bump" any large underlying masses or organs. (12)

24 Sluggish or drowsy behavior. (8)

25 A condition where an unconscious patient does not respond to any stimuli. (4)

26 The sense of a body part position. (14)

28 The first cervical vertebra. (5)

29 Tapping the body's surface to produce vibration and sound. (10)

30 Horizontal __ is described as recurrent flickering back-and-forth eye movements. (9)

31 The site of gas exchange in the lungs. (8)

32 The patient's attentiveness or reaction to its environment. (9)

33 The junction of an axon with another nerve cell. (7)

Down

1 Vertebrae located in the abdominal region; they serve as the site of attachment for the large sling muscles that support the abdomen. (6)

2 To classify patients according to the severity of illness or injury to determine their relative priority for treatment. (6)

3 Flaps of tissue are also known as __. (5)

4 The tail vertebrae are also known as the __ vertebrae. (9)

5 The central nervous system is made up of the __ and spinal cord. (5)

8 An abnormal buildup of cerebrospinal fluid in the brain. (13)

11 The phase of the heart where the heart chambers relax to receive the blood. (8)

14 The basic structural and functional unit of the nervous system. (6)

15 A hollow sound, such as that produced by air-filled lungs. (9)

17 The flap of cartilage that acts as a "trapdoor" to cover the opening of the larynx during swallowing. (10)

18 Using the hands and the sense of touch to detect tenderness, altered temperature, texture, vibration, pulsation, masses or swellings, and other changes in body integrity. (9)

19 A cerebrovascular accident is also called a/an __. (6)

20 An irregular heartbeat. (10)

22 The condition in which a semiconscious patient can respond to noxious (painful) stimuli. (6)

27 The position or carriage of the body. (7)

28 A wobbly or uncoordinated gait. (6)

Chapter **22** **Patient History and Physical Examination**

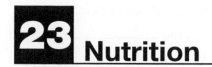

23 Nutrition

After reviewing this chapter, the reader will be able to:
- List basic energy-producing and non–energy-producing nutrients
- Describe considerations for feeding young and adult dogs
- Describe considerations for feeding young and adult cats
- Discuss the fundamentals of exotic pet diet considerations
- Explain nutritional peculiarities of livestock
- Give examples of methods used in feeding livestock
- Discuss basic differences in the digestive tracts of ruminants and monogastric animals

TRUE OR FALSE

1. _____ Allowing livestock to harvest forage avoids costs incurred in mechanical harvesting.

2. _____ Concentrates are generally low in fiber and high in energy and protein.

3. _____ During aspiration of a feeding tube, there should never be negative pressure on the syringe if the feeding tube is placed correctly.

4. _____ It is acceptable for clients to constantly change their cats' diet with various brands and types of commercial diets.

5. _____ Weaning of kittens should begin at 5 weeks of age.

6. _____ Feline urinary tract disease tends to occur more often in obese, sedentary cats.

7. _____ Domestic dogs do not need a variety in their diets.

8. _____ Puppies should begin weaning at 3 to 4 weeks.

9. _____ Many complications of parenteral nutrition involve the catheter.

10. _____ It is acceptable to feed iguanas commercially prepared food.

11. _____ Domestic livestock extract essential nutrients from plant material.

12. _____ Grass hay has a much higher level of protein than alfalfa.

13. _____ Aging diminishes the sense of taste and smell.

14. _____ Force-feeding is preferred because it is a stress-free way to get nutrients into the pet.

15. _____ Iguanas are herbivores.

FILL IN THE BLANK

1. The digestive system converts the food eaten by the animal into _____ that body cells use for metabolic fuel.

2. Water balance in the system affects the ability to excrete _____.

3. Cow's milk is not an acceptable milk substitute for puppies because it contains _____.

4. _____ must be based on age, breed, health status, activity level, and reproductive condition.

5. Allowing pets free access to food at anytime increases _____, which leads to obesity.

6. Pet foods should be tested by this association: _____

7. Sick or injured pets need good nutritional support to counteract the immunosuppressive effects of these five

things: _____, _____, _____, _____, and _____.

8. After feeding tube placement the amount of food is gradually increased over 3 days with 5 ml of water every

_____.

9. These four things are suitable prey for most species of snakes: _____, _____, _____,

and _____.

10. Alfalfa and red and white clover are all _____ commonly used for forage production.

11. The total daily fluid volume for maintenance TPN is _____.

12. Shelf life of vitamin C is _____, not from the date of purchase.

13. Orogastric intubation is excellent for rapid administration, but it can cause _____

and _____.

14. _____ of dextrose is needed to avoid hyperglycemia.

15. Hay should have less than _____ to be stable in storage.

MATCHING

Match the following items to the description on the right.

1. _____ Body-conditioning score

2. _____ Forage

3. _____ Byproduct feeds

4. _____ Herbivore

5. _____ Obesity

6. _____ Portion control feeding

7. _____ Free choice feeding

8. _____ Time control feeding

9. _____ Water

10. _____ Essential amino acids

11. _____ Nonessential amino acids

12. _____ Nutrient

13. _____ Carnivore

14. _____ Water-soluble vitamins

15. _____ Fat-soluble vitamins

A. Amino acid that is synthesized in the body
B. Meat eater
C. Vitamins absorbed from the small intestines—excess amount excreted in urine
D. Vitamins metabolized and stored in the liver
E. Plant eater
F. Method of subjectively qualifying body fat reserves
G. Residues of food-processing industry
H. Daily portion offered either in single feeding or divided into several portions
I. Foundation for metabolism of all nutrients in the body
J. Most common nutritional disorder of pets
K. Feeds made up of most or all plant
L. Access to food 24 hours a day
M. Amino acid that cannot be synthesized in the body
N. Any constituent of food that can be ingested to support life
O. Portion fed with access for only 10 to 15 minutes

1. List the six basic nutrients.

    1. _____,

    2. _____,

    3. _____,

    4. _____,

    5. _____,

    6. _____,

2. Name five dietary minerals discussed in this chapter.

    1. _____,

    2. _____,

    3. _____,

    4. _____,

    5. _____,

3. Describe time-controlled feeding.

    _____,

    _____.

4. List vitamins that may be required in older dogs.

    1. _____,

    2. _____,

    3. _____,

    4. _____,

    5. _____,

5. Obesity may predispose pets to what three things?

    1. _____,

    2. _____,

    3. _____,

6. Describe techniques used to enhance aroma and taste of food for cats.

_____

_____

_____

7. Name three reasons that homemade diets are not always the best for the pet.

_____

_____

_____

8. What does the acronym AAFCO stand for?

_____

9. Total parenteral nutrition is a practical alternative for patients that:

a. _____

b. _____

c. _____

d. _____

10. Describe the method mentioned for adding vitamin C to drinking water.

_____

_____

_____

11. Describe ways to prevent injury or death of a snake when feeding.

a. _____

b. _____

c. _____

12. Describe the diet suggested for box turtles.

_____

_____

13. What do nonnutritive feed stuffs provide?

a. _____, b. _____, c. _____, d. _____, e. _____.

14. List the legumes commonly used for forage.

a. _____, b. _____, c. _____, d. _____, e. _____.

15. Diet selection used in enteral nutritional support is based on:

a. _____

b. _____

c. _____

MULTIPLE CHOICE

1. To break down cellulose, herbivores depend on:
   a. bacteria
   b. microorganisms
   c. parasites
   d. both a and b

2. Energy is used for:
   a. metabolism
   b. fighting disease
   c. skin turgor
   d. clotting

3. Dietary protein is used for:
   a. digestion
   b. metabolism
   c. building body tissue
   d. cell repair

4. Cow's milk is not a proper milk replacer for neonatal puppies. Cow's milk is lacking:
   a. glucose and phosphorus
   b. protein and lactose
   c. potassium and sodium
   d. iron and selenium

5. Diets for active dogs must have enhanced levels of:
   a. magnesium
   b. selenium
   c. fat
   d. phosphorus

6. Phosphorus should be limited in older dogs due to detrimental effects on:
   a. liver
   b. kidney
   c. heart
   d. lungs

7. Prevention of uroliths involves manipulation of the dietary intake of minerals, water, and:
   a. fiber
   b. vitamin A
   c. vitamin C
   d. fat

8. Although canned food has greater palatability than dry food, its use raises some concerns for the health of the:
   a. kidneys
   b. teeth
   c. heart
   d. lungs

9. A patient is a candidate for nutritional support if the animal has:
   a. lost more than 10% of body weight
   b. diarrhea with body conditioning loss
   c. organ dysfunction
   d. all of the above

10. Acceptable routes of nutritional support can include:
    a. enteral
    b. parenteral
    c. intravenous
    d. all of the above

WORD SEARCH

Identify the term described and then find the words in the Word Search.

1. One kind of hay _____

2. Plant-eating animals _____

3. Organic compound made of chains of amino acids _____

4. Nutrient that contains more energy per unit of weight than any other _____

5. Delivery of nutrients directly into the stomach _____

6. Meat-eating animals _____

7. The building blocks of protein _____

8. Any constituent of food that is ingested to support life _____

9. An essential mineral _____

10. The process of converting food into chemical substances that can be absorbed into the blood and used by the body tissues _____

11. Materials of nutritional value fed to animals _____

12. Feed made up of most or all of the plant _____

13. Organic substance found in foods that is essential in small quantities for growth, health, and survival _____

14. That portion of ingested foodstuffs that cannot be broken down by intestinal enzymes and therefore passes through the colon undigested _____

15. Given by injection _____

16. The set of chemical reactions that happen in living organisms to maintain life _____

17. Excessive accumulation of fat in the body _____

18. Energy or power _____

19. A dietary mineral that can have detrimental effects on the kidney _____

20. Organs that filter the blood and excrete the end products of body metabolism in the form of urine _____

```
I  T  A  I  Q  L  A  R  H  L  A  T  O  P  P  U  N  V  W  H
L  L  L  L  A  C  H  R  A  I  M  N  Q  T  L  Q  X  K  E  D
P  U  N  D  F  D  G  R  Z  D  I  E  F  Q  P  R  D  R  M  N
N  H  U  O  F  A  E  Q  R  F  N  I  P  E  M  F  B  Q  N  R
B  W  O  P  I  T  L  R  I  X  O  R  M  N  E  I  J  L  X  J
S  Z  W  S  N  T  E  F  F  C  A  T  B  D  V  D  E  M  R  K
G  P  I  E  P  B  S  Q  A  C  C  U  V  O  T  J  I  G  L  M
O  A  R  X  I  H  D  E  Q  V  I  N  R  L  A  R  E  T  N  E
T  A  B  F  U  V  O  H  G  V  D  E  V  I  T  A  M  I  N  O
P  T  I  S  J  C  A  R  O  I  S  Z  V  K  C  R  D  Q  F  F
Z  N  Z  W  L  F  R  U  U  A  D  Y  Q  F  Y  F  G  A  V  A
W  R  A  G  X  B  R  E  Q  S  O  E  E  N  K  A  D  P  B  T
M  E  T  A  B  O  L  I  S  M  B  G  Y  N  D  T  R  Q  F  K
B  P  F  I  A  Z  K  Z  U  L  E  A  P  E  D  O  W  L  B  Q
E  M  Z  Q  C  N  U  I  W  U  S  R  H  F  T  I  S  Z  Y  U
Q  P  C  T  O  Q  N  W  Z  U  I  O  Q  E  E  N  K  U  U  O
Z  U  X  Z  O  E  X  H  X  U  T  F  I  I  W  V  J  X  S  V
C  V  T  L  L  K  T  R  V  U  Y  N  Y  F  G  T  W  M  N  R
X  V  C  E  F  O  R  C  E  R  O  V  I  N  R  A  C  L  N  Q
B  S  S  I  Q  B  P  E  S  S  I  H  V  D  V  I  G  Q  J  E
```

WORD SCRAMBLE

Unscramble the words below.

1. tetnunri _____
2. rtnepio _____

3. iodgetnsi _____
4. eilnrams _____

5. carsbydathoer _____
6. cirenrvoa _____

7. maeotsbiml _____
8. teyordndiha _____

9. etneral _____
10. nrartepale _____

11. iehrroveb _____
12. eugmle _____

13. pisild _____
14. yaahrdrcebto _____

15. tffdusee _____
16. lesagi _____

17. slrumootc _____
18. uintare _____

19. lebsulo _____
20. pbyiaiilltat _____

CROSSWORD PUZZLE

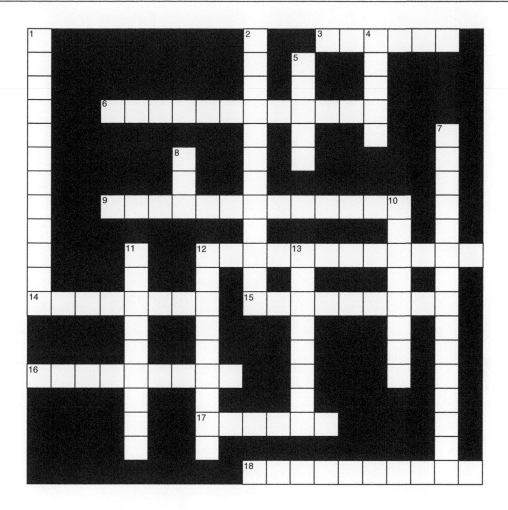

Across

3 A partially fermented forage state. (6)
6 Medication added to feed would be classified as a __ feed additive. (12)
9 __ scoring is a method of subjectively quantifying subcutaneous body fat reserves. (2 words) (13)
12 Microbial __ is the process by which herbivores break down cellulose. (12)
14 Forage harvested at a given stage of development and fed directly. (8)
15 __ amino acids cannot be synthesized in the body and so must be supplied by the diet. (9)
16 The __ analyses are determinations of dry matter (DM), crude protein (CP), ether extract (EE, crude fat), crude fiber (CF), and ash. (9)
17 Feed made up of most of the plant. (6)
18 Energy-producing nutrients have a hydrocarbon structure that produces energy through digestion, __, or transformation. (10)

Down

1 Feeds that are low in fiber and high in energy and/or protein. (12)
2 The __ __ extract is the nonfiber carbohydrate portion of the feed. (2 words) (12)
4 __ -soluble vitamins are metabolized in a manner similar to fats and stored in the __. (5)
5 __ -soluble vitamins are passively absorbed from the small intestine, and excess amounts are excreted in the urine. (5)
7 Agammaglobulinemic animals are born without __. (15)
8 Forage that is cut and allowed to dry before being collected into bales for storage. (3)
10 Any constituent of food that is ingested to support life. (8)
11 The type of feeding where food is offered at all times so the animal can eat at its leisure. (2 words) (9)
12 Any dietary component that provides some essential nutrient or serves some other function. (9)
13 The harvesting process by which forage is chopped and placed into a storage unit that excludes oxygen. (8)

Nursing Care of Dogs and Cats

LEARNING OBJECTIVES

After reviewing this chapter, the reader will be able to:
- Describe techniques used in the general nursing care of dogs and cats
- Discuss techniques used in the recording of patient care
- Describe procedures used in grooming, skin, nail, and ear care
- List common routes of administration of medication and describe procedure used in administration of medications
- List and describe methods of parenteral administration
- List and describe methods of intravenous catheterization
- List and describe methods of urethral catheterization
- List and describe methods of orogastric and nasogastric intubation
- Discuss procedures used in nursing in special circumstances
- Describe methods of respiratory support
- Discuss procedures used in caring for recumbent patients
- Discuss issues related to techniques used in the care of neonatal puppies and kittens
- Discuss issues related to techniques used in the care of geriatric patients

TRUE OR FALSE

1. _____ Lung sounds are more subtle in the dog than the cat.

2. _____ Pulmonary crackles found on auscultation usually indicate severe dehydration.

3. _____ A patient's posture can help assess ventilation efficiency.

4. _____ Presence of a cough usually indicates heart disease in the cat.

5. _____ Buccal or transmucosal administration of medications can be effectively achieved in both the canine and feline patient.

6. _____ A pulse deficit may indicate an arrhythmia.

7. _____ Respiratory sinus arrhythmia is common in dogs, but very uncommon in the cat.

8. _____ Persistent jugular distension is an important indicator of right heart failure.

9. _____ Mild soapy water can be an effective enema solution in the constipated patient.

10. _____ Paradoxical ventilatory patterns and movements may indicate diaphragmatic hernia or some neurologic condition.

SHORT ANSWER

1. What is a common respiratory lung sound auscultated in the asthmatic patient?

_____

2. A French Bulldog presents with labored breathing. Auscultation is difficult due to referred airway sounds. What are some other means to assess ventilation?

_____

_____

_____

3. List some common rule-outs (explanations) for pale mucous membranes; brick-red mucous membranes?

_____

_____

4. What is a physiologic murmur?

_____

5. Characterization of a heart murmur can be based on the PMI. What does this acronym stand for? Why is it important?

_____

_____

6. What is the difference between vomiting and regurgitation? Why is this clinically important?

_____

_____

_____

7. a. Why is it important to characterize any abnormal stools in a patient's medical record?

_____

_____

   b. What is included in a visual stool analysis?

_____

   c. Why is dietary history important in terms of stool quality?

_____

   d. How can the technician monitor GI motility?

_____

8. A geriatric dog presents to your clinic with the complaint of ataxia and a head tilt. What neurologic assessments should be performed by the technician as part of the physical exam?

_____

_____

9. During a physical exam of a dog with a history of lethargy, you note small pin-point red dots on the ventral abdomen. The mucus membranes are pale.

   a. What could this be indicative of?

_____

   b. What pertinent questions should be asked of the owner?

_____

c. What are the general nursing concerns with this dog?

_____

d. What would be the most logical site for venipuncture?

_____

10. A dog with a history of vaccine reactions presents for his yearly exam. The owner insists on vaccinations despite potential complications because they are moving to a state where vaccines are mandatory.

a. What are the common signs of a vaccine reaction?

_____

b. What preventive measures can be taken prior to vaccinations?

_____

c. If a reaction occurs, what is the treatment of choice?

_____

d. If anaphylaxis occurs, what is the standard treatment?

_____

11. A Great Dane is recovering from spinal surgery for a ruptured cervical disc. His vitals are as follows: T = 97.0, HR = 200, R = 79, MM are pale, and pulse quality IS poor.
Auscultation is difficult over shivering and growling.

a. What are some possible explanations for the elevated heart rate?

_____

_____

b. What are some possible reasons for the increased respiratory rate?

_____

_____

c. What could explain poor pulse quality?

_____

_____

d. What are some explanations for pale mucous membranes?

_____

_____

e. The dog will not be able to walk for several days. What is standard protocol for any recumbent patient?

_____

_____

f. Are there any special considerations regarding a recumbent Great Dane?

_____

_____

12. Pain control is a high priority in the field of veterinary nursing.

    a. List some common signs of pain in the small animal.

_____

_____

    b. What are some physiologic consequences of pain?

_____

_____

    c. Other than analgesia administration, what are some ways of providing comfort to the patient?

_____

_____

MULTIPLE CHOICE

1. Typical signs of dehydration include:
   a. bradycardia
   b. hypersalivation
   c. inelasticity of skin
   d. pale mucous membranes

2. Common signs of catheter-related phlebitis include:
   a. pitting edema
   b. limb numbness
   c. cold extremity
   d. limb atrophy

3. Most sick neonates experience:
   a. hyperthermia
   b. hypoglycemia
   c. vomiting
   d. hypoxia

4. Which of the following is not typically used to treat severe hypothermia?
   a. intravenous fluids
   b. electric heating pads
   c. circulating water pads
   d. warm water bottles

5. Contraindications to epidural injections include:
   a. patients with coagulation disorders
   b. geriatric patients
   c. dehydrated patients
   d. pediatric patients

6. Which intravenous solutions listed below are recommended to be administered through a central line?
   a. hypertonic or hyperosmolar solutions such as partial parenteral nutrition
   b. blood products
   c. colloid solutions
   d. crystalloid solutions only

7. Decubital ulcers typically form in which location?
   a. tail tip
   b. bony prominences such as the femur
   c. oral cavity
   d. ocular regions only

8. Signs of anal gland impaction include:
   a. excessive water intake
   b. vomiting
   c. anorexia
   d. scooting of the hindquarters

9. The measurement of the force of the blood exerted during the relaxation phase, when the aortic and pulmonic valves are closed, is called:
   a. diastolic blood pressure
   b. mean arterial pressure
   c. systolic blood pressure
   d. capillary wedge pressure

10. Level of consciousness is an important vital sign because it can:
    a. be an indicator of CNS abnormalities.
    b. determine whether a patient has an infection.
    c. be an indicator of ocular abnormalities.
    d. assess a patient's need for IV fluids.

11. Daily weighing is of particular importance in patients receiving:
    a. antibiotics
    b. chemotherapy
    c. large amounts of intravenous fluids
    d. enteral nutrition

12. Pulse deficits may indicate:
    a. dehydration
    b. sepsis
    c. inflammation
    d. arrhythmias

13. A normal respiratory sinus arrhythmia has a normal to slow heart rate and is characterized by:
    a. an increase in heart rate during inspiration and a decrease in heart rate during expiration
    b. a decrease in heart during inspiration and an increase in heart rate during expiration
    c. absolutely no effect with expiration or inspiration
    d. an effect with expiration only

14. Auscultation should be to performed with the patient in:
    a. right lateral recumbency
    b. left lateral recumbency
    c. sternal recumbency
    d. any body position because sounds do not vary with patient position

15. Respiratory distress that is exacerbated by recumbency is termed:
    a. dyspnea
    b. tachypnea
    c. orthopnea
    d. cyanosis

16. Enemas are contraindicated if:
    a. the bowel is distended
    b. recent colon surgery has been performed
    c. vomiting occurs
    d. the patient is dehydrated

17. Medications that can be introduced through the nasal passages include:
    a. general anesthetics
    b. antibiotics
    c. respiratory vaccines
    d. analgesics

18. Inspiratory dyspnea almost invariably indicates:
    a. an upper airway disorder
    b. cardiac disease
    c. asthma in the feline patient
    d. fluid overload

19. Before administration of any ocular medication:
    a. ensure the eye is not cloudy
    b. remove any excess hair or debris that may deter application
    c. provide excessive restraint
    d. ensure blink response is present

20. SQ fluids are contraindicated in which of the following?
    a. vomiting
    b. dehydration
    c. shock
    d. fever

1.

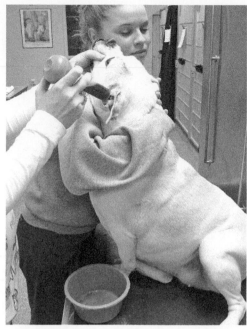

a. Why is it necessary to first examine the ears before medication administration?

_____

_____

b. What are the complications of this procedure if there was damage to the membrane?

_____

_____

c. What are some common clinical signs of ear disease?

_____

_____

2.

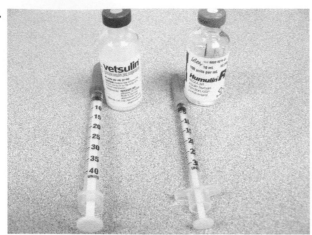

a. What are some important aspects of insulin and insulin syringes that must be relayed to clients.

_____

_____

b. Are there special storing considerations and/or administration tips related to insulin?

_____

_____

c. How important is a routine insulin administration schedule?

_____

_____

d. Is insulin administered before or after a meal?

_____

_____

e. What are the typical signs of hypoglycemia?

_____

_____

3.

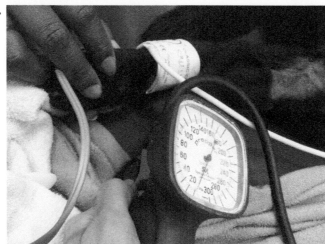

a. What procedure is being performed in the photo above?

_____

_____

b. This device provides which pressure reading?

_____

_____

c. Why is cuff size so important in obtaining accurate measurements?

_____

_____

d. What should be an approximate cuff width in relation to limb circumference?

_____

_____

e. How is the cuff positioned in relation to the artery?

_____

_____

f. How should the patient's body be positioned?

_____

_____

g. Which limb is preferred during measurement, and how can different limbs affect blood pressure values?

_____

_____

4.

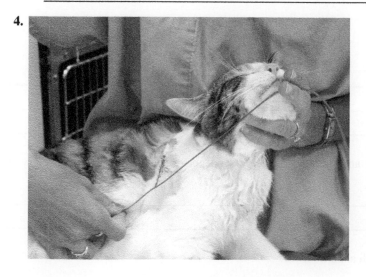

a. What procedure is being performed?_____

b. Why is the tube being held alongside the cat?

_____

_____

c. After the tube is inserted to the premeasured space, why is it immediately aspirated?

_____

_____

d. If excessive air is obtained upon aspiration, what does this mean and what should be done?

_____

_____

e. What are some of the other methods to ensure correct tube placement?

_____

_____

f. Is there any diagnostic step to ensure 100% that the tube is in the correct location?

_____

_____

5.

a. What is the technician doing?

_____

_____

_____

b. Name the abnormality that can be detected and the test that should be performed once that abnormality is detected

_____

_____

c. What are some common explanations for such abnormalities?

_____

_____

6.

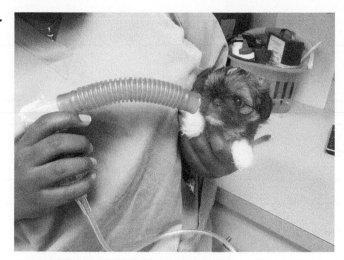

a. What treatment is being performed?

_____

b. What is the goal of this therapy?

_____

_____

c. Why is this patient being held sternal?

_____

_____

d. What is usually performed immediately after this treatment and why?

_____

_____

7.

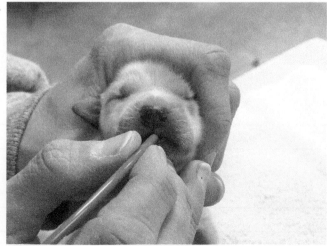

a. What is being performed?

_____

Chapter **24** **Nursing Care of Dogs and Cats**

b. When is this necessary in the neonate?

_____

c. When is this contraindicated?

_____

_____

d. After feeding, what is the proper way to remove the tube?

_____

_____

e. What are some common complications of tube feeding?

_____

_____

f. What is the typical way to assist eliminations? How often and for how long?

_____

8.

a. What procedure is being performed?

_____

_____

b. When is this procedure necessary?

_____

_____

c. Why is this type of catheter being used?

_____

_____

d. What are some common complications when this type of catheter is used?

_____

_____

e. Is this a sterile procedure?

_____

_____

f. Is this the best type of catheter for indwelling use? Why or why not?

_____

_____

g. Why is it usually necessary to place a collection system onto a urinary catheter?

_____

_____

h. What are some common clinical signs of an obstructed cat?

_____

_____

MATCHING

Match the disease or injury below with the proper nursing response from the list below. Choose only one answer per situation.

1. _____ Diabetes mellitus

2. _____ Hepatic lipidosis

3. _____ Renal failure

4. _____ Respiratory distress

5. _____ Seizures

6. _____ Head trauma

7. _____ Spinal trauma

8. _____ Addison's disease

9. _____ Heartworm disease

10. _____ Hit by car

A. monitor for deep pain sensation
B. nutritional intake
C. aggressive fluid therapy
D. establish IV access
E. blood glucose
F. electrolyte analysis
G. serial PCV/TS
H. avoid excessive IV fluid resuscitation
I. strict exercise restriction post treatment
J. oxygen therapy

269

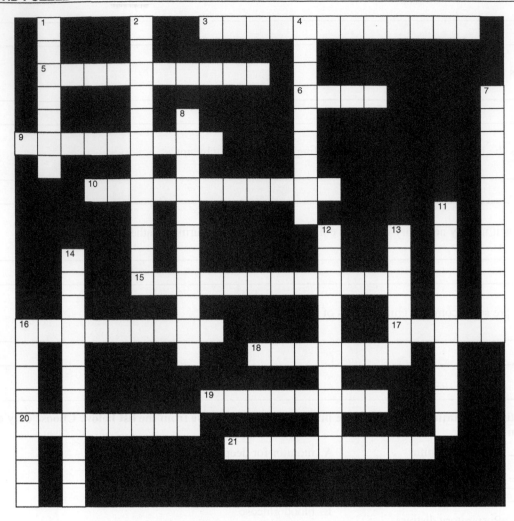

Across

3 Referring to a route of injection directly into the marrow of the bone. (12)

5 A condition in which the eyes are not properly aligned with each other. (10)

6 Systolic blood pressure is the maximum force caused by contraction of the __ ventricle of the heart. (4)

9 A/an __ ulcer is a pressure sore exacerbated by recumbency, increased skin moisture, and irritation. (9)

10 Acute and severe multisystemic hypersensitivity reaction. (11)

15 Normal body temperature. (12)

16 Local venous inflammation. (9)

17 Suspension of external breathing. (5)

18 The __ venous pressure is the pressure within the cranial vena cava monitored by catheterization of the cranial vena cava via the jugular vein. (7)

19 Straining to defecate. (8)

20 An increase in the concentration of deoxygenated hemoglobin, characterized by blue mucous membranes. (8)

21 Involuntary eye movement. (9)

Down

1 Increased respiratory effort or difficulty breathing. (7)

2 Humidification of inspired gases to promote mobilization and removal of unwanted secretions in patients with respiratory disease. (12)

4 Pain relief, in the form of oral, transdermal, or injectable medication. (9)

7 Abnormally slow heart rate. (11)

8 Abnormally fast heart rate. (11)

11 The act of ending a patient's life in a humane manner. (10)

12 An abnormal heart rhythm. (10)

13 Referring to the cheek. (6)

14 The lack of gas exchange within alveoli, usually due to alveolar collapse or fluid consolidation. (11)

16 Small red or purple spots on the body, caused by minor hemorrhage or broken capillary blood vessels. (8)

Nursing Care of Horses

LEARNING OBJECTIVES

After reviewing this chapter, the reader will be able to:
- Discuss the principles of feeding, watering, exercising, and bedding of horses
- Explain and demonstrate routine procedures used in grooming and foot care
- Discuss the techniques used in general nursing care of horses
- Identify specific nursing procedures used in caring for recumbent horses
- Discuss the methods of sample collection for laboratory analysis
- State the pros and cons of using various routes of administration of medication
- List the steps necessary for the proper intravenous catheterization of horses

COMPLETE THE CHART

Write in the most appropriate feed for a horse with the particular disease or condition listed in the right column.

Feed	Disease or Condition
	Chew and swallow normally
	Impactions
	Diarrhea
	Allergies or pneumonia
	GI ulcerations
	Oral lesions or hoking
	Neuromuscular, botulism

List the four sites that an IM injection can be given on the horse in the first column; then list an appropriate safety technique if using that site.

Muscle/Site	Safety Technique

FILL IN THE BLANK

1. Horses require _____ gallons of water daily.

2. _____ shavings are not acceptable bedding for horses with open wounds or respiratory disorders.

3. Black walnut shavings can cause _____ when the horse stands in the shavings.

4. Recumbent adult horses must have very deep bedding to help prevent formation of _____

   _____ .

5. Fly sprays containing _____, _____, or _____ are the safest for sick horses.

6. _____ currycombs should not be used on the horse's head or distal limbs.

7. _____ appears as black, malodorous material in the region of the frog.

8. Antibiotic therapy can develop into life-threatening diarrhea from changes in bowel _____.

9. Nonsteroidal antiinflammatory drugs for an orthopedic problem can cause _____ _____ or _____ _____.

10. Critically ill neonates require frequent monitoring, as often as every _____ hours.

11. Recumbent animals must be turned frequently to prevent _____ _____ on the skin and _____ and _____ in the lungs.

12. If a horse requires assistance to stand, the hind limbs can be supported by suspending a rope attached to the _____ from a ceiling beam.

13. A sling cannot be used for horses with _____ _____.

14. A topical spray that creates a _____ bandage may provide the best protection for decubital ulcers.

15. Food and water may have to be given by _____ tube to a recumbent animal.

16. Care must be taken to avoid wrapping tape over the _____ _____ because excessive pressure can reduce circulation to hoof tissues, causing damage or sloughing of the hoof.

17. The _____ vein is the most commonly used vein to obtain blood samples from a horse.

18. In seriously ill horses an alternative to the jugular vein is the _____ _____, which is ventral to the facial crest.

19. A horse that cannot chew or swallow normally can be fed and hydrated through a _____ tube.

20. If the nasogastric tube strikes the ethmoturbinates as it pasts through the pharynx, the _____ _____ may bleed profusely.

21. The adult horse's stomach can hold _____ to _____ liters, but can vary between horses.

22. _____ should be administered intravenously only because it can be very caustic and cause tissue sloughing.

23. No more than _____ ml of solution should be given to mature horses in one IM site.

24. The _____ is the only appropriate vein for IV injections in horses.

25. Medications inadvertently injected into the carotid artery pass directly to the brain and can cause severe _____, _____, and even _____.

26. _____ catheters can be left in the vein for 3 to 5 days if the insertion site is kept clean and there is no sign of swelling or thrombophlebitis.

27. _____ or _____ catheters can be left in the vein for up to 2 weeks if adequate care is used in preserving the catheter.

28. The injection plug and IV tubing should be changed every _____ hours because bacteria may proliferate within the lines.

29. Horses with endotoxemia, any type of gastrointestinal disorder, or Gram-negative infections are at the highest risk of forming a _____.

30. Critically ill neonates are often _____, so IV fluids should be warmed to body temperature before infusion.

31. Plasma is stored frozen and requires thawing in _____ _____, NOT in the _____.

32. Blood transfusions should be considered when the hematocrit falls below _____% to _____%.

33. Plasma, serum, and blood should be infused slowly, giving _____ to reduce the chance of an adverse reaction.

34. Special IV administration sets that contain a filter to catch any _____ _____ are necessary when administering plasma or blood products.

35. Severe _____ _____ may require topical treatments as often as every 1 to 2 hours.

SHORT ANSWER

1. Explain why getting a starting weight on a horse or foal when admitted to the hospital is so important.

_____

_____

_____

_____

2. Describe how to roll a recumbent adult horse.

_____

_____

_____

_____

3. Describe the steps involved in wrapping the distal part of a horse's leg.

_____

_____

_____

_____

4. Describe how to wrap a tail on a horse using a long plastic sleeve.

_____

_____

_____

_____

5. List three things to check to be certain the nasogastric tube is not inserted into the trachea?

1. _____

_____

2. _____

_____

3. _____

_____

6. Explain the proper technique for removing a nasogastric tube from the horse's stomach.

_____

_____

_____

_____

7. What two emergency drugs should be on hand in case of anaphylactic shock?

_____

_____

8. Provide the direction in which the IV catheter should be lying inside of the following veins:

Jugular

_____

_____

Cephalic

_____

_____

Lateral thoracic

_____

_____

Saphenous

_____

_____

9. List five signs of an adverse reaction to blood or plasma infusions.

1. _____

2. _____

3. _____

4. _____

5. _____

Identify the term described and then find the terms in the Word Search.

1. Materials used to provide comfort, conservation of body heat, protection of bony prominences, and ease of cleaning _____

2. A structure in an ultrasound image that appears bright or white compared with adjacent structures _____

3. Rapid breathing _____

4. A destructive metabolic process by which complex substances are converted by living cells into simpler compounds, with release of energy _____

5. Abnormally low body temperature _____

6. Inflammation of a vein associated with clotting _____

7. Severe abdominal pain of sudden onset caused by a variety of conditions, including obstruction, twisting, and spasm of the intestine _____

8. Abnormally low circulating blood volume _____

9. Degenerative condition of the hoof that may occur secondary to a bacterial infection and appears as black, malodorous material in the region of the frog _____

10. Pressure sores (bedsores) that result from an animal lying on a bony prominence for too long _____

11. An uncommon, complex disorder of newborns that results from a blood group incompatibility between mother andoffspring that causes the destruction of the offspring's RBCs _____

12. A local defect produced by sloughing of necrotic inflammatory tissue _____

13. Gap between teeth, as seen between incisors and cheek teeth of some species _____

14. Inflammation of the hoof lamina; also called founder _____

15. Wheal formation on the skin; commonly referred to as hives _____

16. Difficulty eating _____

17. Pertaining to the nose and stomach, used particularly to describe placement of a feeding tube into the stomach via the nares _____

18. Difficulty breathing _____

19. Compounds that are commonly used as insecticide dips and may result in toxicity if used inappropriately

_____

20. Delicate bony scrolls located in the nasal cavity of some species _____

21. Pertaining to "around a blood vessel" _____

22. Any disease of the stomach and intestines _____

23. Inflammation of the lungs with tissue consolidation _____

```
B  S  A  C  A  D  W  N  L  L  V  I  P  X  I  F  A  H  E  S  B  Z  I  D  L
E  B  L  N  F  G  X  G  U  K  E  Q  O  E  R  T  Y  M  U  O  J  Y  S  O  K
W  U  U  L  V  A  Y  U  W  E  G  Y  M  H  R  P  B  S  E  E  Z  O  M  L  M
E  K  O  T  T  P  M  Y  U  F  A  O  I  L  E  I  T  E  A  T  E  R  E  Z  Z
A  E  N  P  Y  H  C  A  T  I  Y  J  X  R  T  T  V  T  I  E  S  L  Z  Q  K
S  E  I  H  T  A  P  O  R  E  T  N  E  O  R  T  S  A  G  M  A  A  G  O  A
J  P  B  Q  Q  K  D  L  L  O  D  C  Y  W  N  B  U  H  S  Q  K  X  I  X  I
C  R  S  I  E  G  D  A  R  Y  H  C  T  I  J  S  L  P  G  C  J  J  S  D  R
H  I  O  I  A  U  T  J  S  O  V  W  T  S  S  N  A  S  N  O  U  T  A  B  A
P  A  M  Y  T  I  L  P  I  Z  Y  H  O  E  E  A  M  O  I  P  I  L  Z  P  C
O  N  U  R  B  I  H  C  O  E  A  Y  T  W  H  S  I  H  D  U  U  C  A  L  I
Y  R  E  U  E  A  B  Q  E  O  P  A  C  V  Z  O  N  P  D  F  W  M  W  R  T
F  E  C  U  G  H  Y  E  S  R  N  K  O  T  B  G  I  O  E  E  U  J  Z  E  R
W  E  M  I  M  C  T  A  L  I  S  V  L  D  H  A  T  N  B  F  B  Y  L  A  U
D  C  A  S  U  O  E  O  B  H  K  B  I  Z  J  S  I  A  T  H  R  U  S  H  W
M  P  G  D  D  N  N  R  P  V  P  H  C  E  Y  T  S  G  Q  B  J  A  S  C  M
B  T  A  D  P  G  U  I  W  Y  V  O  L  K  N  R  V  R  V  F  J  M  G  X  S
Q  P  X  S  W  T  X  F  A  F  H  X  B  K  X  I  I  O  V  W  D  G  S  O  E
Z  G  Y  Z  O  Z  T  P  J  Z  I  D  W  M  G  C  Q  D  M  W  M  W  V  O  R
Q  D  M  M  Q  I  S  O  E  R  Y  T  H  R  O  L  Y  S  I  S  L  T  H  B  V
R  I  H  A  I  M  E  L  O  V  O  P  Y  H  X  R  U  Q  K  Z  X  L  V  S  C
H  T  I  F  W  I  F  U  L  X  Y  O  O  M  R  H  H  Z  P  H  O  A  F  Q  E
E  C  A  T  A  B  O  L  I  C  I  B  Z  U  B  P  O  T  T  C  V  U  I  T  V
G  C  M  Y  F  L  A  W  I  Q  Q  J  S  X  X  V  Y  S  G  O  P  P  I  P  A
W  B  V  F  Y  L  E  Y  O  G  C  M  N  E  J  Y  N  B  C  O  J  R  B  R  I
```

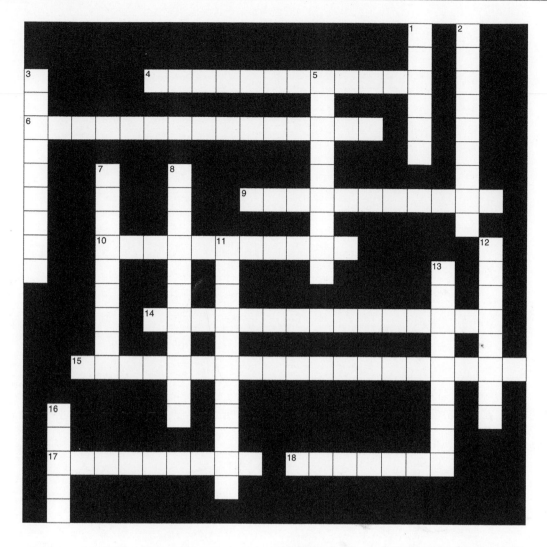

Across

4 Pertaining to "around a blood vessel." (12)
6 Delicate bony scrolls located in the nasal cavity of some species. (15)
9 Abnormally low circulating blood volume. (11)
10 Abnormally low body temperature. (11)
14 An uncommon, complex disorder of newborns that results from a blood group incompatibility between mother and offspring that causes the destruction of the offspring's RBCs. (15)
15 Diseases of the stomach and intestines. (19)
17 Inflammation of the hoof lamina; also called *founder*. (9)
18 Difficulty breathing. (7)

Down

1 Degenerative condition of the hoof that may occur secondary to a bacterial infection and appears as black, malodorous material in the region of the frog. (6)
2 Wheal formation on the skin; commonly referred to as *hives*. (9)
3 Inflammation of the lungs with tissue consolidation. (9)
5 A destructive metabolic process by which complex substances are converted by living cells into simpler compounds, with release of energy. (9)
7 Rapid breathing. (9)
8 Pertaining to the nose and stomach, used particularly to describe the placement of a feeding tube into the stomach via the nares. (11)
11 A structure in an ultrasound image that appears bright or white compared with adjacent structures. (11)
12 Gap between teeth, as seen between incisors and cheek teeth of some species. (8)
13 Difficulty eating. (9)
16 Severe abdominal pain of sudden onset caused by a variety of conditions, including obstruction, twisting, and spasm of the intestine. (5)

Across

26 Nursing Care of Food Animals, Camelids, and Ratites

LEARNING OBJECTIVES

After reviewing this chapter, the reader will be able to:
- Explain general husbandry terms and techniques used with food animals and ratites
- Compare and contrast various routes of administration of medication in food animals and ratites
- Explain the techniques used in general nursing care of food animals and ratites
- Identify and describe various methods of sample collection for laboratory analysis
- State the steps necessary for the proper procedure for intravenous catheterization
- Demonstrate proper procedures used in grooming and foot care

MATCHING

Select the proper male or female name for the following animals.

1. _____ Adult intact male ovine

2. _____ Male adult bovine

3. _____ Young caprines

4. _____ Adult female porcine

5. _____ Young camelid

6. _____ Adult intact male caprine

7. _____ Castrated male porcine

8. _____ Female adult bovine

9. _____ Castrated male ovines/caprines

10. _____ Adult female caprine

11. _____ Male castrated bovine

12. _____ Young ovine

13. _____ Female young adult bovine

14. _____ Young porcine

15. _____ Intact adult male porcine

16. _____ Adult female ovine

17. _____ Young female porcine before farrowing

A. Gilts
B. Bull
C. Piglets
D. Doe
E. Lambs
F. Sow
G. Heifer
H. Buck/ram
I. Boar
J. Cria
K. Kids
L. Billy/ram
M. Steer
N. Ewe
O. Barrow
P. Wether
Q. Cow

COMPLETE THE CHART

Select the appropriate needle or indwelling catheter sizes for the animals listed below.

Animal Species	IM Injection	SC Injection	IV Injection	IV Blood Draw	IV Catheter
Cow					
Goat					
Sheep					
Newborn Calf/Lamb/Kid					
Pig					
Piglet					
Llama					

Needle Sizes: 14, 16, 18, 20, 22, 23, 25, 26 gauge

Needle Lengths: ⅜, ⅝, ¾, 1, 1.5, 2, 3, 4, 6 inch

Catheter Sizes: 14 ga × 2 inch   16 ga × 2 inch   18 ga × 2 inch   20 ga × 2 inch   22 ga × 2 inch

16 ga × 6 inch   18 ga × 6 inch   20 ga × 6 inch

FILL IN THE BLANK

1. The gestation period for cattle is about _____ months.

2. Many beef and almost all dairy operations now use _____ with frozen bull semen as a common method of breeding.

3. Gestation for sheep and goats is about _____ months.

4. The procedure for removing wool from around the vulva and udder on sheep is called _____ or
_____.

5. The major use of goats today is for _____ and _____ production.

6. The gestation period for swine is approximately _____ months, _____ weeks, and _____ days.

7. The newborn piglet has eight very sharp canine teeth referred to as _____ teeth.

8. The best time to castrate male piglets is before _____ weeks of age.

9. Minimum length of time that must pass from the last administration of a medication until the time the animal is

slaughtered or the milk is collected for human consumption is referred to as _____ _____.

10. Boluses (large tables), capsules, or magnets may be given per os (PO) with a _____ _____.

11. A balling gun with a large, _____ head will produce less trauma to the pharyngeal tissue but is easily damaged by teeth.

12. In food animals, the stomach tube is usually passed through the _____ cavity, with the aid of a metal speculum.

13. When vaccinating an entire herd of cattle, a/an _____ _____ syringe will do the job more efficiently.

14. ID injections of tuberculin are most often given in the _____ tail fold.

15. The common reaction to an intranasal insufflation is _____.

16. Employ intramammary infusions to treat _____ or to infuse _____ quarters when cows are not lactating.

17. When performing intrammary infusion, do not insert the cannula to the hub because this stretches the _____ _____ and predisposes the quarter to _____.

18. Medication is placed in the uterus to locally treat _____.

19. A sterile sleeve should be worn to insert _____ or _____ into the uterus.

20. It is difficult to catheterize male goats and bulls because of the _____ diverticulum at the ischial arch.

21. Jugular venipuncture requires that the animal is _____ and restrained in a chute or stanchion

22. In pigs blood is usually collected from the _____ vein or the _____ vena cava.

23. The _____ vein is most often chosen for IV catheterization in food animals.

24. Indwelling catheters can be left in place for _____ days.

25. Hydraulically operated "tilt tables" are made specifically for _____ _____, making the task safe and efficient.

26. The _____ is the largest of the four species of camelids.

27. When placing a halter on a llama, you should avoid _____ eye contact.

28. A vaccination program for camelids should include _____ _____ and _____.

29. The young camelids that are infested by _____ suffer from diarrhea.

30. Castration of camelids is usually performed after _____ years of age.

31. The _____ muscles are avoided in camelids when giving an IM injection, so it is given in the _____ and _____ muscles.

32. _____ rheas are the most aggressive of the three common species.

33. Intramuscular injections are usually given in the _____ muscles over the rump and in the proximal thigh.

34. Needle and catheter sizes for blood sampling of ratites are _____ and _____ gauge.

SHORT ANSWER

1. Describe how to place a balling gun down a cow's throat to deliver a bolus.

_____

_____

_____

2. Describe how you would measure how far down to place a stomach tube regardless of size or species of animal.

_____

_____

_____

Chapter **26** **Nursing Care of Food Animals, Camelids, and Ratites**

3. Describe how you can check to make sure a stomach tube went down the esophagus on a ruminant.

_____

_____

_____

4. What should you do if you see blood aspirated into a syringe before giving an IM injection?

_____

_____

_____

5. Give the maximum volume of medication that can be given in each location:

	IM	SC
Calf/Sheep/Goat	_____	_____
Adult Cow	_____	_____
Pig	_____	_____

6. What three veins are most commonly used for venipuncture in each location:

_____

_____

_____

7. Of the veins used for IV injections which one is the most apt to thrombose and/or roll?

_____

_____

_____

8. Which two animals have accessible auricular veins?

_____

_____

_____

9. What hazard is associated with an intraperitoneal injection?

_____

_____

_____

10. Describe how to check if an IV catheter is still in place.

_____

_____

_____

11. What two species of camelids are considered domesticated?

_____

_____

_____

12. How many compartments does a camelid stomach have?

_____

_____

_____

13. Why is it difficult to perform an IV injection or catheterization on a llama?

_____

_____

_____

14. What vessel can be inadvertently punctured when doing a blood draw on a camelid?

_____

_____

_____

15. What vein is accessible on crias that is similar to dogs?

_____

_____

_____

16. The term ratite refers to what type of animal?

_____

_____

_____

17. Unthrifty plumage on a ratite may indicate what conditions?

_____

_____

_____

18. Give the TPR values expected from a ratite.

_____

_____

_____

19. What special considerations are needed when restraining ratites?

_____

_____

_____

20. Describe how to "hood" a ratite.

_____

_____

_____

WORD SEARCH

Identify the term described and then find the words in the Word Search.

1. A large tablet or ball of food that is intended to be swallowed or a large amount of fluid or liquid medication given quickly, intravenously (as opposed to being given slowly— "titrated") _____

2. Pregnancy: the state of being pregnant; the period from conception to birth when a female animal carries a developing fetus in her uterus _____

3. Washing cells from the air sacs at the end of the bronchioles _____

4. A space, void of teeth, found in both the upper and lower arcades and extends from the corner incisors to the first premolars _____

5. The round, muscular structure that separates the uterus (cranially) from the vagina (caudally) _____

6. The minimum length of time that must pass from the last administration of the medicine until the time that the animal is slaughtered for food or the milk is collected for human consumption _____

7. The production and secretion of milk by the mammary glands _____

8. Those vertebrae found in the tail _____

9. A South American camelid, widely used as a pack and meat animal by Andean cultures _____

10. A fluid-filled, raised area on the surface of the skin that is the result of an allergic or hypersensitivity reaction to an irritant or a small, but palpable, amount of fluid that was injected into the top layers of the skin by using a syringe and a small-gauge needle _____

11. Thin, yellow fluid that is the first milk produced by the breast in the first few days after delivery _____

12. A flexible tube that is passed through the mouth (oro-), down the esophagus, and into the stomach (-gastric) for the purpose of delivering fluids and liquid medication directly into the stomach _____

13. The place where two things are joined _____

14. The surface region between the pubic bone and the tail bone _____

15. The removal of wool from around the tail and between the rear legs of a sheep _____

16. A dairy cow that is not being milked during her dry period. The dry period usually consists of a 60-day window between the end of one lactation cycle and the expected birth of another calf, which will start a new lactation cycle _____

17. Around or surrounding a blood vessel _____

18. Procedure in which the vein is exposed surgically and then a cannula is inserted into the vein under direct vision _____

19. Giving birth _____

20. An area of dense tissue that replaces the upper incisors in most ruminant species _____

21. Gravity flow IV system used to administer fluids to large animals _____

22. Giving small volumes of liquids PO _____

23. A category of non flying birds _____

Chapter 26 **Nursing Care of Food Animals, Camelids, and Ratites**

```
I Y Z S A W P D I O V S U M D D V V Q J R H D L I
B S F O T D D C P A R T U R I T I O N A R E A N R
N R U J Y F B O M Q K D Y Q J D R J L M H E T B B
N U O L R C I C E B T C Q T V Q N U O C H E C I H
O X C N O Y F C F M O D J M B V C O T W R W E P B
I E X N C B F Y E W I A B H C S A U I D A X R Y M
T Y O E M H Y G U X L T Z Y A W R N E T C X V G U
A E F G H Q O E J E O X L V L C Q N G M A V I G J
T P E R I A N A L U L D I A X Y T X C Z Y T X H X
C Y D U S W Q L L W X R D M W A Q C O P H H S N G
A D Q I R L X V M V E B B Z L A E T I T A R T E L
L K M U C I W E E P E G C S Y H R H R X U R Y Y G
J B O D B H C R T G X O P O T B I D A Q W S Q P A
B I C L E X Y T S K O A L C M G N I H C N E R D M
A J O A V P P E Y V C Z P A S M O R B T T N D C A
R O L M T X V B S E G B I M R R I U G V I S W B L
R S O M M V B R X F A A L R L L W S Q V D W U K L
Q K S M I W S A E T C F Q J C H A Z S E V N Y R K
I D T J M S M E L J Y U H A C X D V N U T J P R G
M R R L I U P H P C N J T Q P R J T A L R Z K T P
P M U W P A B S M M J S G D U U A P J G F E K E K
B K M V V E H V I F C L T M O L M B X G E Q D C R
E B U T C I R T S A G O R O P W P V R H B A T F W
E V R R J K Q W S C W O T A W A N C N O C S M Q F
I V H O T E M O D G U H D M D V F N L O G C A I U
```

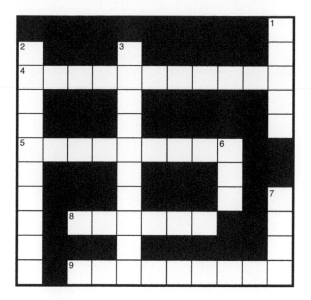

Across

4 The __ space is a space, void of teeth, found in both the upper and lower arcades and extends from the corner incisors to the first premolars. (11)

5 An area of dense tissue that replaces the upper incisors in most ruminant species. (2 words) (9)

8 The round, muscular structure that separates the uterus (cranially) from the vagina (caudally). (6)

9 The vertebrae found in the tail. (9)

Down

1 A large tablet or ball of food that is intended to be swallowed OR a large amount of fluid or liquid medication given quickly, intravenously. (5)

2 The __ time is the minimum length of time that must pass from the last administration of the medicine until the time that the animal is slaughtered for food or the milk is collected for human consumption. (10)

3 The __ tube is a flexible tube that is passed through the mouth down the esophagus and into the stomach for the purpose of delivering fluids and liquid medication directly into the stomach. (10)

6 A __ cow is a dairy cow that is not being milked during the 60-day window between the end of one lactation cycle and the expected birth of another calf which will start a new lactation cycle. (3)

7 A fluid-filled, raised area on the surface of the skin that is the result of an allergic or hypersensitivity reaction to an irritant OR a small, but palpable, amount of fluid that was injected into the top layers of the skin by using a syringe and a small gauge needle. (5)

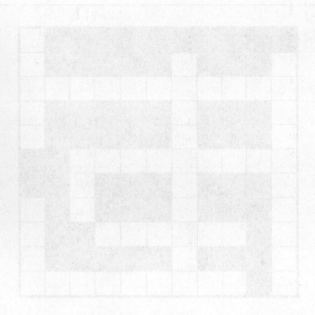

Nursing Care of Companion Birds, Reptiles, and Amphibians

LEARNING OBJECTIVES

After reviewing this chapter, the reader will be able to:
- Describe the unique features of the anatomy of birds and basic biology of common reptile species
- Discuss the basic behavior of birds, reptiles, and amphibians
- Discuss the basics of client education, husbandry, and nutrition for the avian, reptile, and amphibian species
- Describe how to obtain a complete and thorough history of the avian, reptile, and amphibian patient
- Explain the different capture and restraint techniques used for birds, reptiles, and amphibians
- Identify methods of sample collection for laboratory analysis
- Describe how to obtain quality diagnostic images of avian reptile and amphibian patients
- Discuss nursing care & supportive therapy techniques for the avian, reptile, and amphibian patient
- Identify and discuss some of the common diseases and presentations of the avian, reptile and amphibian patient to the veterinary clinic
- List the common infectious diseases and zoonoses found in the avian, reptile, and amphibian patient
- Describe the routine clinical procedures performed on avian, reptile, and amphibian species
- Explain the unique aspects of avian, reptile, and amphibian anesthesia and surgery
- Identify and discuss some of the common presentations, emergencies, & critical care

LABEL

Identify the elements in this right lateral view of a psittacine.

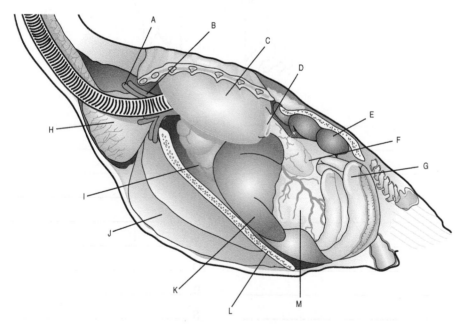

A. _____

B. _____

C. _____

D. _____

E. _____

F. _____

G. _____

H. _____

I. _____

J. _____

K. _____

L. _____

M. _____

Identify the elements in this ventrodorsal view of the psittacine.

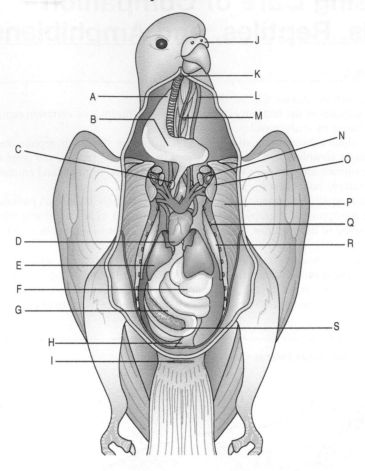

A. _____

B. _____

C. _____

D. _____

E. _____

F. _____

G. _____

H. _____

I. _____

J. _____

K. _____

L. _____

M. _____

N. _____

O. _____

P. _____

Q. _____

R. _____

S. _____

MATCHING

Match the anatomic term on the left with the description on the right.

1. _____ Anisodactyl
2. _____ Coprodeum
3. _____ Coracoid
4. _____ Coverts
5. _____ Proctodeum
6. _____ Pygostyle
7. _____ Remiges
8. _____ Supracoracoideus
9. _____ Urodeum
10. _____ Uropygial
11. _____ Zygodactyl

A. Caudal part of the cloaca
B. Cranial portion of the cloaca that receives feces from the rectum
C. A platelike bone at the distal vertebrae, consisting of fused caudal vertebrae
D. Middle part of the cloaca; most of the bird
E. Another term for large primary flight feathers
F. A paired bone part of the shoulder
G. Arrangement of feet with second and third toes facing forward and the first and fourth toes directed backward
H. Located at the end of the pygostyle
I. Arrangement of feet so that three toes point forward and one toe points to the rear
J. Body feathers that provide surface coverage over
K. The muscle ventral to the pectorals

SHORT ANSWER AND FILL IN THE BLANK

1. What are some principles that should be kept in mind when feeding avian species:

   1. _____
   2. _____
   3. _____
   4. _____
   5. _____

2. Signs of respiratory distress in a bird include:

   1. _____
   2. _____
   3. _____
   4. _____
   5. _____
   6. _____
   7. _____
   8. _____

3. Hydration can be assessed by:

   1. _____
   2. _____
   3. _____
   4. _____
   5. _____

Chapter **27** **Nursing Care of Companion Birds, Reptiles, and Amphibians**

4. Signs of egg retention include:

   1. _____

   2. _____

   3. _____

   4. _____

   5. _____

   6. _____

5. What signs should you watch for when determining if a bandage needs to be changed?

   1. _____

   2. _____

   3. _____

   4. _____

6. Common signs of anesthesia that can be noted visually include:

   1. _____

   2. _____

   3. _____

   4. _____

7. For the administration of fluid and medication in lizards:

   1. It is best to use the _____ site if the gastrointestinal tract is effective.

   2. The most common sites are usually the _____ and _____. Because of the _____, only the _____ should be used.

   3. The route rarely used is the _____.

   4. Sedation or equivalent would be required if the _____ route is utilized.

   5. Use the _____ route for administration of fluids where the patient is best placed in _____ recumbency. It is important to _____ prior to administering any fluids.

8. List at least 10 basic anesthetic supplies and pieces of equipment that would be needed for reptile patients:

   1. _____

   2. _____

   3. _____

   4. _____

   5. _____

   6. _____

   7. _____

   8. _____

   9. _____

   10. _____

9. What are some ways to minimize future behavior problems for parrots?

_____

_____

_____

_____

_____

_____

10. Where should the Doppler probe be placed for obtaining a heart rate in the following species?

Lizards _____

Snakes _____

Chelonians _____

Amphibians _____

11. List the common venipuncture sites for the following species:

Chelonians _____

Lizards _____

Snakes _____

12. List the common intravenous catheter sites for the following species:

Chelonians _____

Lizards _____

Snakes _____

TRUE OR FALSE

1. _____ The average adult bird has a core body temperature of 38 to 42.5° C (105 to 112° F).

2. _____ If a blood feather needs to be removed, it should be pulled in the direction opposite to the way it is growing.

3. _____ When flushing a wound, care needs to be taken that the puncture is not communicating with an air sac.

4. _____ The uropygial gland is absent in the ostrich, emu, cassowaries, bustards, frogmouth, many pigeons, woodpeckers, and Amazon parrots.

5. _____ Since birds have complete cartilaginous tracheal rings that cannot expand, inflated cuffed tubes are best used. Manual ventilation, high oxygen flow rates, and high-pressure ventilation are safe to use.

6. _____ The proventriculus, or true stomach, is very similar to the stomach of mammals, containing digestive acid and enzymes.

7. _____ The largest muscles in the avian body are the pectorals.

8. _____ Grit is required in the gizzard to properly digest hard foods.

9. _____ When a bird is stressed, there is an increased fecal component to the droppings because they pass before lower intestinal water resorption occurs.

10. _____ In most birds ovulation to egg laying takes approximately 15 hours.

11. _____ Birds' circulatory systems differs from those of mammals in that the red blood cells of birds are oval and contain a nucleus; but birds do have lymph nodes.

Chapter **27** **Nursing Care of Companion Birds, Reptiles, and Amphibians**

12. _____ To minimize behavior problems in cockatoos, it is best to repeatedly pet the bird over its back and tail.

13. _____ To properly capture birds, towels should be used as much as possible while gloves and bare hands should be discouraged.

14. _____ A good place to capture a bird is from the owner's shoulders.

15. _____ The best time to examine a bird is when the crop is full.

16. _____ To help prevent passive reflux of barium into the mouth during a gastrointestinal contrast study, a small vetwrap bandage can be placed round the bird's neck close to the mandible.

17. _____ When using a Dremel® to beak trim cover the nares as you hold the beak shut.

18. _____ The general rule of wing-trim is that the heavier the bird, the fewer primary and secondary feathers are to be removed.

19. _____ If a bird is to be microchipped, anesthetize and aseptically prepare the pectoral muscle site.

20. _____ Use greasy or oily medications or silver sulfadiazine topically for avian burns.

21. _____ Wood that should not be used for perches includes black locust, oak, and rhododendron.

22. _____ When anesthetizing birds, start at a low percentage of the gaseous anesthetic and increase until the desired depth of anesthesia is reached.

23. _____ Birds do not show signs of seizuring.

24. _____ Snakes generally shed their outermost skin in pieces. Prior to a shed the skin and eyes become opaque. Handling should be kept to a minimum at this time.

25. _____ Box turtles have hinged plastrons, so the easiest way to extend their heads is by gently propping open the cranial portion of the carapace and the plastron.

26. _____ Keeping one hand on the neck, just behind the base of skull, will help prevent getting bitten when handling long-necked lizards.

27. _____ Subcutaneous fluids are commonly given into the inguinal or axillary region of chelonians.

28. _____ Contrary to belief, daily soaking of reptiles will not help improve overall hydration.

29. _____ Urine is not concentrated in the kidneys in birds; rather urine moves retrograde into the coprodeum and rectum, where resorption of water, sodium, and chloride takes place.

30. _____ Amazon parrots are the only species that will develop hematuria in acute cases of heavy metal toxicosis.

31. _____ When examining a turtle, a clinician can place one or two fingers in the inguinal area between the hind limbs and the shell to palpate the coelomic cavity.

32. _____ In order to examine the cloacal mucosa properly, it must be everted and all four quadrants of the cloaca must be examined.

33. _____ When surgically preparing a bird, all feathers, including flight feathers, should be removed by pulling in the direction of the growth.

34. _____ Alcohol is the agent of choice when flushing the dilute chlorhexidine from a surgical site.

35. _____ Most diseases in exotic animals are caused by poor husbandry and improper diet.

36. _____ Male iguanas and bearded dragons have very large femoral pores as compared to females.

37. _____ Many species of male tortoises have a concave plastron, making it easier to mount the female.

38. _____ The probe used to determine a snake's sex will advance further into the cloaca of a female snake.

39. _____ EDTA is the anticoagulant used for chemistry evaluation while lithium heparin is the anticoagulant generally used for CBC evaluation in birds and reptiles.

40. _____ To obtain an accurate core body temperature during avian anesthesia, the clinician should place an esophageal temperature probe as far as the proventriculus.

MULTIPLE CHOICE

1. With reference to the respiratory system of birds:
   a. Air enters through the nares and continues over an operculum.
   b. An epiglottis is present.
   c. Lobes and alveoli are present so the lungs can inflate.
   d. The diaphragm assists inspiration of air through extension of the intracostal joints.

2. Regarding airflow in birds:
   a. Birds have a total of five paired air sacs.
   b. The unpaired air sac is the interclavicular air sac.
   c. The respiratory tract cannot communicate with the long bones.
   d. Gas exchange occurs in the air sacs.

3. Regarding special senses of birds, which statement is not true?
   a. Birds have the traditional five senses: seeing, hearing, feeling, smelling, and tasting.
   b. The vision and hearing control centers are larger than those for taste, touch, and smell.
   c. Birds have very acute vision and can perceive color.
   d. Birds have a good sense of taste.

4. With regards to avian anesthesia:
   a. Birds should be fasted 10 to 12 hours prior to anesthesia.
   b. The crop should be empty to prevent aspiration.
   c. Routine use of parasympatholytic agents such as atropine and glycopyrrolate are routine.
   d. Benzodiazepines such as diazepam and midazolam have analgesic properties.

5. With regards to reptilian anesthesia:
   a. Premedications are given intramuscularly caudal to the kidneys.
   b. Premedication needs to be given only 20 minutes prior to anesthetic induction.
   c. Propofol is the most common injectable induction agent used in reptiles.
   d. Lactated Ringer solution is usually given at a rate of 50 ml/kg/h.

6. Regarding reptilian biology:
   a. Like birds, reptiles have a diaphragm to separate the thoracic and abdominal cavities.
   b. There is one visceral cavity called the coelom.
   c. Most reptiles do not have a renal portal system.
   d. Reptile excrement contains two components—urates and feces.

7. Which statement is true regarding nutrition and feeding?
   a. Chicken breast, hot dogs, and raw beef provide a complete diet for snakes.
   b. Lizards are usually only herbivores.
   c. Most aquatic turtles are omnivorous.
   d. Tortoises are omnivores and eat a variety of leaves, grasses, and insects in the wild.

8. With the physical examination, which statement is incorrect?
   a. The kidneys of lizards sit in the pelvic girdle and are palpated via rectal examination.
   b. Septicemia of iguanas is noted as petechiae and ecchymosis on dorsal spines.
   c. Generally, there is a narrow range of normal physiologic values in reptiles.
   d. Heart rates vary depending on temperature, age, species, and health status.

9. How much blood can safely be taken from a 700-g healthy lizard?
   a. 70 ml
   b. 56 ml
   c. 7.0 ml
   d. 5.6 ml

10. When examining or restraining amphibians:
    a. It is not necessary to wear nonpowdered vinyl or latex gloves when handling.
    b. Keep the patient dry when handling to avoid dehydration.
    c. One hand should support the body near the pelvis.
    d. Organs are easily palpated.

11. Regarding husbandry of reptiles:
    a. The only purpose of cage furniture is to provide a hiding place.
    b. Hot rocks and sizzle stones can cause thermal burns.
    c. Any ultraviolet (UV) lighting will assist reptiles with synthesizing vitamin D.
    d. The green iguana requires decreased levels of humidity to stay healthy.

12. With amphibian care or feeding:
    a. Temperature, pH, salinity, and water hardness should be checked on a regular basis.
    b. Nitrogenous waste buildup and disinfectant residues are easily tolerated.
    c. Alkalinity, dissolved oxygen, and nitrate need not be checked on a regular basis.
    d. Most amphibians are herbivores as adults.

13. When performing a venipuncture of amphibians:
    a. Alcohol is best used to clean the venipuncture site.
    b. Venipuncture in salamanders is generally performed using the caudal tail vein.
    c. A 20- to 22-gauge needle attached to a 1.0-ml syringe should be used.
    d. The femoral and lingual veins are commonly used in frogs and toads while the ventral abdominal vein is the most difficult.

14. What is the MER for a 20-g canary?
    a. 6.7
    b. 10.05
    c. 7.5
    d. 12.5

15. What is the maintenance fluid rate for 24 hours for an 85-g nondehydrated cockatiel?
    a. 42.5 ml
    b. 22.5 ml
    c. 4.25 ml
    d. 2.25 ml

MATCHING

1. _____ Avian polyomavirus (APV)

2. _____ Chlamydiosis

3. _____ Lead and zinc

4. _____ Poxviruses

5. _____ Proventricular dilatation
disease (PDD)

6. _____ Psittacine beak and feather
disease (PBFD)

7. _____ *Salmonella* spp.

8. _____ West Nile virus

A. Seen as early as 10 weeks of age in African grey parrots, cockatoos, and conures
B. Psittacines appear to be somewhat resistant to this mosquito-borne virus
C. Most often associated with imported Amazons and macaws
D. Easily spread by feather dust, dander, and feces to other birds
E. Intermittently shed by reptiles if they are carriers of this bacteria
F. Two heavy metals most commonly encountered with avian patients
G. Zoonotic disease that causes psittacosis in humans
H. Most common viral cause of death in budgerigar breeding facilities

PLACE IN PROPER ORDER

Intraosseous catheter placement of avian patients

1. _____

2. _____

3. _____

4. _____

5. _____

6. _____

7. _____

8. _____

9. _____

A. Insert the cannula just above the dorsal condyle of the distal ulna.
B. Wrap the wing with a figure eight bandage.
C. Suture the cannula into place.
D. Flush with heparinized saline.
E. Grasp the ulna with one hand and insert the cannula with the other.
F. Cap off the cannula with a sterile infusion plug.
G. Remove the stylette.
H. Pluck a few feathers over the dorsal, distal ulna, and surgically prep the area.
I. Advance the cannula into the medullary cavity.

DEFINITION

Define the acronyms below.

1. POTZ _____

2. ECG _____

3. IPPV _____

4. PBFDV _____

5. WNV _____

6. PMV-3 _____

7. OSHA _____

8. BMR _____

9. MER _____

Chapter **27** **Nursing Care of Companion Birds, Reptiles, and Amphibians**

Define the terms below.

1. Pneumatic: _____

2. Synsacrum: _____

3. Operculum: _____

4. Coprodeum: _____

5. Diurnal: _____

6. Pygostle: _____

7. Avulsion: _____

8. Dysecdysis: _____

9. Petechiae: _____

10. Ecchymosis: _____

11. Kyphosis: _____

12. Celiocentesis _____

PICTURE QUIZ

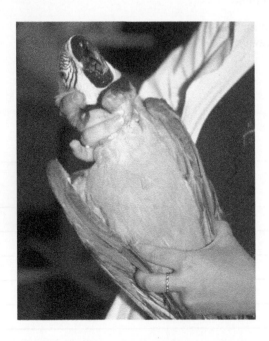

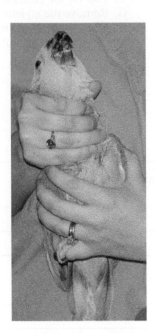

1. Is this hold of this bird correct? Why or why not?

_____

_____

2. Is this the correct restraint for this parrot? Why or why not?

_____

_____

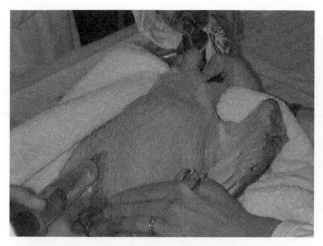

3. The site for these subcutaneous fluids is _____, which is the site of choice because _____. Use a _____ -gauge needle.

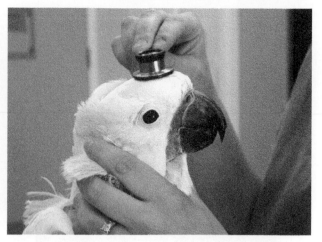

4. What is the purpose of auscultating the top of the head?

_____

_____

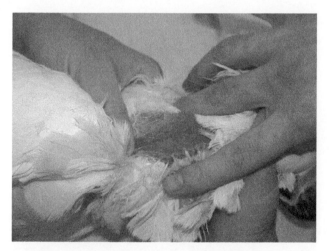

5. Is this site appropriate for a small bird?

_____

_____

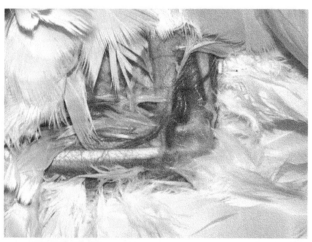

6. Why should the _____ not be used routinely for blood collection?

_____

_____

Chapter **27** **Nursing Care of Companion Birds, Reptiles, and Amphibians**

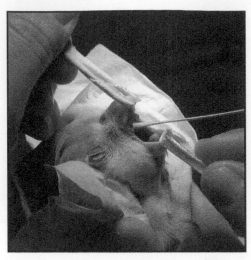

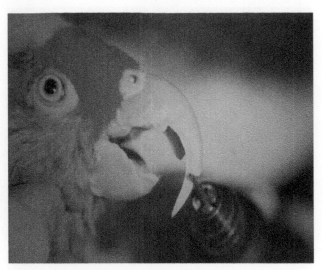

7. What procedure is being performed, and what is the best restraint for a bird of this size?

_____

_____

8. The instrument used to trim this beak is

a _____. Do not cover the

_____ when restraining the beak.

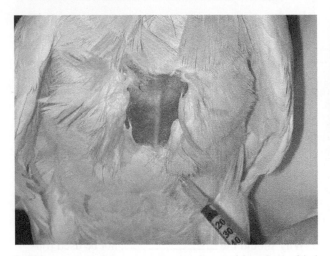

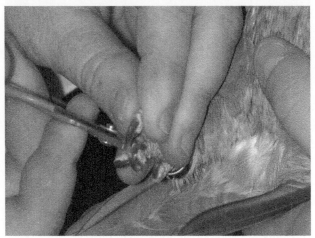

9. Use no more than _____ ml in a large bird

in this _____ IM site.

10. Why are regular nail trims important?

_____

_____

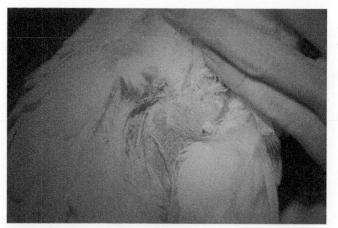

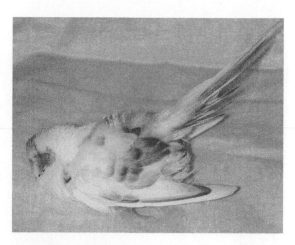

11. The cause of crop fistula in this hand-fed juvenile cockatoo is likely. _____

12. This bird is showing signs of. _____

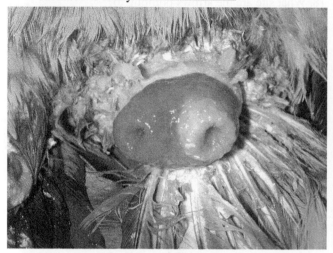

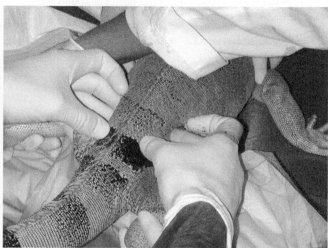

13. The most important immediate therapy for prolapsed cloaca is _____.

14. What area is being palpated in this iguana?

_____

_____

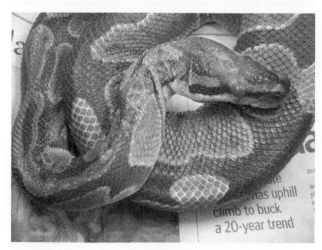

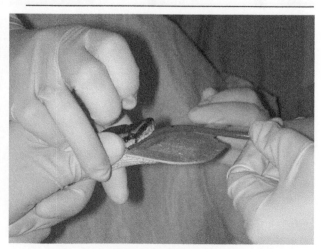

15. This snake's skin and eyes are turning an opaque, blue color. What is happening?

_____

_____

16. What procedure is being completed in this picture? Is the device used correct?

_____

_____

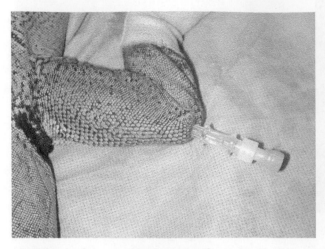

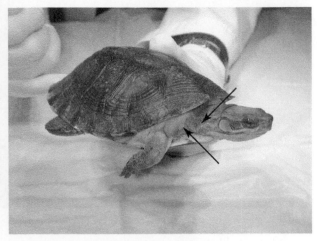

17. What is the procedure being performed and what are some precautions?

_____

_____

18. What site are the arrows pointing to?

_____

_____

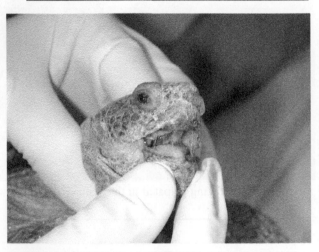

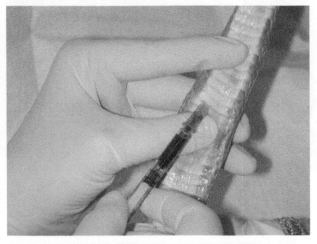

19. What are signs of severe dehydration in reptiles?

_____

_____

20. For cardiocentesis in a snake, where should the needle be specifically located?

_____

_____

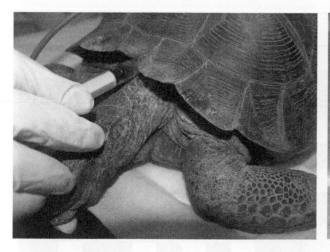

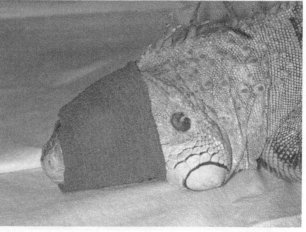

21. What site is being used, and how is the blood obtained?

_____

_____

22. What is the purpose of the cotton balls over the eye and an elastic wrap?

_____

_____

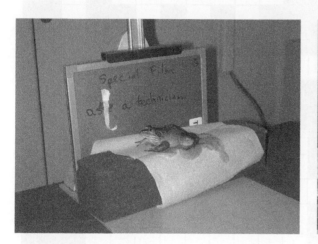

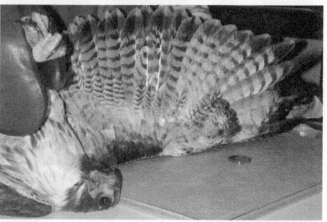

23. What view is being taken?

_____

_____

24. What view is being prepared?

_____

_____

Chapter **27** **Nursing Care of Companion Birds, Reptiles, and Amphibians**

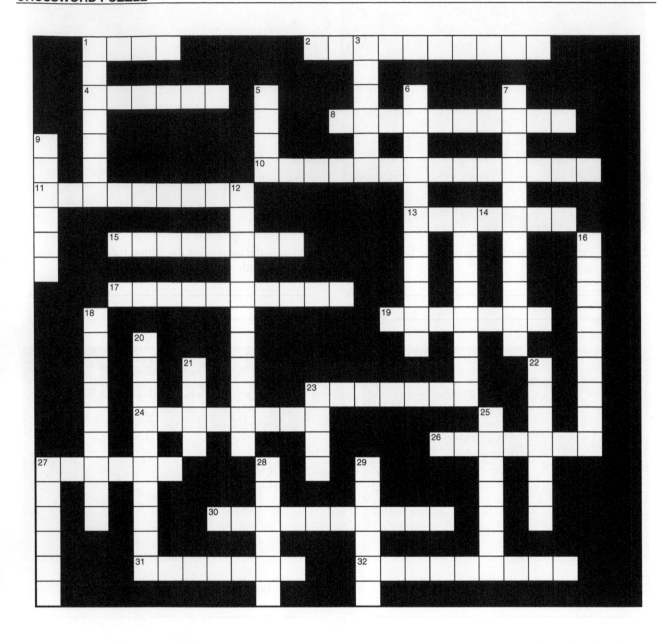

Chapter **27** **Nursing Care of Companion Birds, Reptiles, and Amphibians**

Across

1 The __ feathers are a layer of fine feathers under the exterior feathers. (4)
2 The feet psittacines that are shaped so that the second and third toes face forward with the first and fourth toes directed backward. (10)
4 The end product of nitrogenous waste production from the liver that is excreted by the kidney as a pasty white-to-yellow material found in bird droppings. (6)
8 Perching birds and songbirds such as canaries, finches, and sparrows. (10)
10 The glandular portion of the stomach responsible for production of the gastric juices and propulsion of food into the ventriculus (gizzard). (14)
11 The middle ear bone in birds. (9)
13 Nine thin, transparent membranes that are connected to the primary and secondary bronchi and act as reservoirs for air entering and leaving the lungs. (2 words) (7)
15 A term used to describe a juvenile parrot using the tongue to explore surfaces. (8)
17 The caudal part of the cloaca that empties contents into the vent. (10)
19 Contour feathers found on the wing of a bird; the flight feathers. (7)
23 These feathers are smaller feathers that cover the remiges and rectrices. (7)
24 Feather tracts on the skin of birds. (8)
26 The middle compartment of the cloaca, which is the terminal end to the ureters and genital ducts. (7)
27 The body cavity in birds that extends from the first thoracic rib to the vent. (6)
30 The oral cavity of birds. (10)
31 The process of feather replacement that occurs one to several times a year, depending on the species. (7)
32 Pertaining to species that forage and hunt at night. (9)

Down

1 Pertaining to those species that forage or hunt in the daytime. (7)
3 Feeding with a feeding tube passed through the oral cavity into the stomach. (6)
5 The dilatation of the esophagus located at the base of the neck just cranial to the thoracic inlet. (4)
6 Parrots, macaws, and parakeets. (11)
7 Filled with air. (11)
9 A dark ribbon like structure attached to the retina and extending into the vitreous humor; thought to provide nourishment to the eye. (6)
12 The foot of passerines with three toes that point forward and one toe that points to the rear. (11)
14 Contour feathers found on the tail of a bird. (8)
16 A keratinized flap of tissue inside the nares of some birds. (9)
18 The __ gland secretes a lipoid sebaceous material that is spread over feathers during preening to help with waterproofing. (9)
20 The terminal end of the rectum in the cranial compartment of the cloaca. (10)
21 The bony ridge on the sternum of birds where the flight muscles attach. (4)
22 The featherless areas of birds where there are no feather tracts. (7)
23 The fleshy colored skin located at the base of the upper beak in many bird species. (4)
25 The __ feathers are the largest feathers that form the external appearance of adult birds. (7)
27 The terminal end for the reproductive, urinary, and gastrointestinal tracts. (6)
28 The V-shaped notch in the roof of the mouth of birds that provides communication between the nasal cavity to the oropharynx. (6)
29 The voice box of birds. (6)

28 Nursing Care of Orphaned and Injured Wild Animals

LEARNING OBJECTIVES

After reviewing this chapter, the reader will be able to:
- Discuss ways to provide nursing care of wildlife
- Discuss regulations and laws concerning wildlife care
- Discuss appropriate ways to take a thorough history
- Describe ways to perform a physical examination
- Assess the condition of orphaned or injured wild animals
- Discuss ways to provide supportive care to wild animals
- Describe methods of sample collection and diagnostic testing for laboratory analysis
- Describe how to obtain diagnostic imaging of wildlife
- Identify routes of administration of medication
- Discuss the ethical treatment and releasability of wild animals
- Identify potential zoonotic and infectious diseases in common wild animal species
- Describe the proper use of personal protective equipment

TRUE OR FALSE

1. _____ If a fledgling or hatchling is touched by humans, the mother birds will abandon it.

2. _____ Under many circumstances, a permit is required to work with or possess native wildlife, especially those that are endangered, threatened, or are protected under the Migratory Bird Act.

3. _____ Depending on the species you are working with, general anesthesia may be needed to perform a complete physical examination.

4. _____ To capture a bird, place a towel over the patient, gain control of the head, pin the wings to the body, and pick the patient up.

5. _____ Towels are not useful to capture wild hares and rabbits.

6. _____ It is acceptable to pick up any species of lizard by the tail.

7. _____ Some lizards such as geckos have extremely delicate skin that can easily be damaged by capture and restraint.

8. _____ When being handed a pillowcase that contains a snake, it is not important to first find the snake's head and then gently grasp it from the outside of the pillowcase.

9. _____ Although chelonians are usually the easiest to capture, they are the hardest to restrain.

10. _____ To keep control of the head of a chelonian, it is best to position your thumb on one side of the cranial portion of the neck and the rest of your fingers just behind the base of the skull.

11. _____ Snapping turtles will not actually bite, and if they do, they will not cause serious harm.

12. _____ When performing a physical examination on birds or reptiles, it is a good idea to covertly evaluate the species if possible to view signs of illness that may be hidden.

13. _____ As with the physical examination of dogs and cats, use a systematic approach, starting at the head and working your way down to the tail, and obtaining both a heart and respiratory rate as soon as the animal is removed from the cage.

14. _____ For an oral examination of rodents and rabbits, sedation or general anesthesia may still be required even with the use of a mouth speculum and light source.

15. _____ The same system used to assess body score in dogs and cats may be used with wild mammals, with 9 out of 9 being emaciated and 1 out of 9 being grossly obese.

16. _____ A visual precapture and restraint physical examination is not necessary in wild animals to determine the animal's attitude and mentation before it has been potentially stressed by handling.

17. _____ A systemic infection or sepsis will not be evident on the plastron of a turtle or the dorsal spines of a snake.

18. _____ Most reptile patients can easily be auscultated with a stethoscope.

19. _____ In most species of snake, the heart is located in the center one third of the body.

20. _____ Depending on the species common collection and diagnostic testing for laboratory analysis include fecal flotation, impression smears, Gram stain, nasal flush, and tracheal lavage.

21. _____ Obtaining blood from a severely trimmed toenail is acceptable in birds.

22. Snakes tubes work well for radiographing snakes only if the tubes are of appropriate size, making it impossible for the snake to move or become obliqued.

23. _____ It is not uncommon for healthy snakes to have pale mucus membranes.

24. _____ The goal of wildlife medicine should be to treat the species regardless of whether the patient is releasable and able to thrive in the wild.

25. _____ Injectable drugs such as ketamine, dexmedetomidine, xylazine, telazol, full mu opioids, buprenorphine, butorphanol, and midazolam can be used alone or in combination with each other to sedate or induce anesthesia.

DEFINITION

Define the terms below.

1. Autotomize: _____

2. Rhinotheca: _____

3. Chelonian: _____

4. Auscultate: _____

5. Dermatophytes: _____

6. Ectoparasites: _____

7. Tympanum: _____

8. Hemostasis: _____

9. Intracoelemic: _____

10. Intraosseous: _____

11. Herbivore: _____

12. Omnivore: _____

FILL IN THE BLANK

1. Regarding the safety of personnel when handling wild animals or birds:

   a. Personal protective equipment that should be worn includes:

      i. _____

      ii. _____

      iii. _____

      iv. _____

b. Disposable equipment should be considered _____ and be _____.

c. Nondisposable items such as lab coats and goggles should be _____.

d. When removing contaminated protective equipment, _____, _____. Immediately after

_____.

e. The most important way to prevent the spread of disease is _____.

2. When force-feeding orphaned birds:

a. Hatchlings should be fed every _____ minutes.

b. Nestlings should be fed every _____ minutes.

c. Fledglings should be fed every _____ minutes.

d. Juveniles should be fed every _____ hours.

e. Birds may not eat at every feeding, but you should still _____.

3. With regards to fluid therapy of orphaned and injured patients:

a. If raptors and nonraptors are not eating on their own, the fluid of choice is often _____. This is

generally given via the _____ route, in the _____ area at a rate of _____ ml/kg/day.

b. Mammals generally have a slightly higher rate when fluids are administered at _____ ml/kg/day, while

the maintenance fluid rate of reptiles tends to be lower at _____ ml/kg/day.

MULTIPLE CHOICE

1. For venipuncture of small birds:
   a. Use the more prominent left jugular.
   b. The bird is best restrained in right recumbency.
   c. A 3-ml syringe with a 25-gauge needle is best.
   d. Hemostasis must be applied to prevent hematomas.

2. To most efficiently obtain blood from a snake:
   a. Perform a cardiocentesis.
   b. The palatine vein is best utilized.
   c. The caudal tail vein is effective in small snakes.
   d. A 10-ml sample volume can easily be obtained.

3. When taking a blood sample from a lizard:
   a. Use the ventral abdominal vein.
   b. The cephalic vein is best.
   c. The ventral coccygeal vein is most effective.
   d. The jugular vein is easily accessible.

4. In a turtle or tortoise:
   a. The radial humoral plexus sinus is generally used in larger chelonians.
   b. The subcarapacial venous sinus is the site routinely used.
   c. If drawing blood from the jugular vein, the turtle/tortoise should be placed in dorsal recumbency.
   d. When drawing blood from the dorsal venous sinus, the patient should be placed in sternal recumbency.

5. Regarding the collection of blood samples:
   a. A Microtainer® is designed for large samples and so is not effective for birds.
   b. Heparin is best used in most species to prevent clumping and staining artifacts of cells.
   c. A larger plasma yield can be achieved by using a Microtainer® containing lithium heparin.
   d. EDTA Microtainers® produce a fibrin clot, immobilizing some of the valuable serum used for sampling.

6. For a sick bird weighing 800 g, what is the suggested maximum safe sample size of blood that should be withdrawn?
   a. 80 ml
   b. 40 ml
   c. 4 ml
   d. 3.2 ml

7. The best views for diagnostic imaging in a chelonian are:
   a. DV, vertical CrCd, and vertical lateral
   b. DV, horizontal CrCd, and horizontal lateral
   c. views in sternal and lateral recumbency
   d. VD and horizontal lateral

8. In avian species, IM injections are best given:
   a. In any muscle mass that is large enough
   b. Cranial to the kidneys
   c. Caudal to the kidneys
   d. Not at all

9. In small mammals:
   a. A subcutaneous injection is usually given over the lumbar region.
   b. A regular needle is preferred over the use of a butterfly catheter for subcutaneous injections.
   c. A 19- to 27-gauge needle can be used based on the size of the patient.
   d. Intramuscular injections are commonly given in the cervical neck muscles.

10. When administering fluids to reptiles:
    a. The patient should be placed in lateral recumbency with the hind leg extended away from the body for an intra-coelomic route.
    b. Intraosseous fluids are not viable in most lizard species.
    c. Intraosseous fluid administration does not require sedation or analgesia.
    d. A spinal needle is placed in the proximal portion of the femur or humerus in lizards.

11. Regarding the nutrition of reptiles:
    a. Carnivorous lizards should be fed whole prey without the bones.
    b. Herbivores should be offered a variety of both dark leafy greens and insects.
    c. Most aquatic turtles are herbivorous, eating only algae and leafy greens.
    d. Do not feed dog food, tofu, monkey biscuits, or anything with animal protein.

12. Raccoons are:
    a. Carriers of *Balisascaris procyonis,* an intestinal roundworm that is zoonotic
    b. Not carriers of *Trypanosoma cruzi*, *Rickettsia rickettsii*, or *Leptospira* sp.
    c. Not susceptible to contracting canine and feline distemper
    d. Disease free, so it is not necessary to wear protective equipment when handling

13. Signs of dehydration in reptiles that can be observed on physical examination include:

    a. A capillary refill time between 1 and 2 seconds

    b. Moist and slimy mucous membranes

    c. Sunken eyes and lack of skin turgor

    d. Tenting of skin that falls immediately

MATCHING

_____ 1. Botulism

_____ 2. Bubonic plague

_____ 3. Bumblefoot

_____ 4. Chlamydiosis

_____ 5. *Cryptosporidium parvum*

_____ 6. *Giardia*

_____ 7. Hantavirus pulmonary syndrome

_____ 8. Lead poisoning

_____ 9. Leptospirosis

_____ 10. Rabies

_____ 11. Salmonellosis

_____ 12. Trauma

_____ 13. Tularemia

_____ 14. West Nile virus

_____ 15. Zinc toxicity

A. Human symptoms include fever, headaches, weakness and vomiting

B. Highly virulent for domestic rabbits and humans

C. Exists in virtually all wildlife droppings with several serotypes being pathogenic to humans and other animals

D. Caused by ingestion of matter left by fishermen or guns

E. Occurs from ingesting galvanized metal or some coins

F. Caused by *Yersinia pestis*

G. The most common presentation for nonraptorial birds

H. Parasite

I. A mosquito-borne disease

J. A zoonotic intracellular bacterial organism

K. This virus causes acute encephalitis and eventual death

L. Affects the plantar surface on the feet of avians in captive management

M. Rodents such as rats and mice are the primary vectors of viruses in this group

N. Etiologic agent is *Clostridium botulinum*

O. Protozoa

PICTURE QUIZ

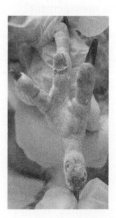

1. What signs are exhibited in this picture?

_____

_____

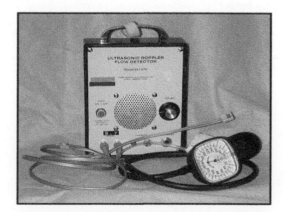

2. What is this instrument, and why is it used?

_____

_____

Chapter **28** **Nursing Care of Orphaned and Injured Wild Animals**

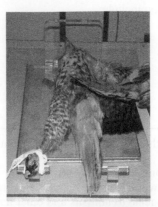

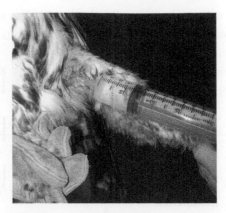

3. What view is this? What is the purpose of the restraint board?

_____

_____

4. What injection site is utilized in this picture?

_____

_____

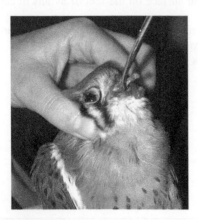

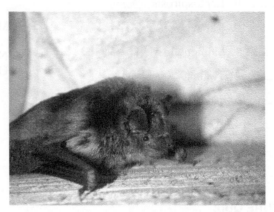

5. What type of feeding tube is generally used in crop feeing birds?

_____

_____

6. What signs are evident in this picture, and why is it a problem of captive management?

_____

_____

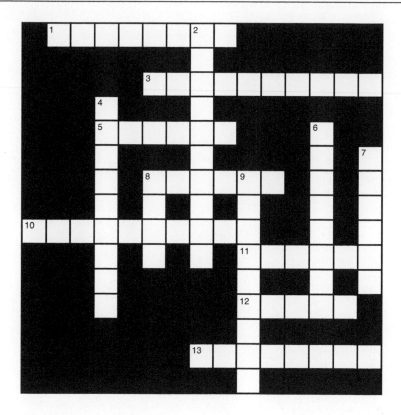

Across

1 An oil-producing gland in a bird used to waterproof feathers. (9)
3 The upper beak of a bird, turtle, or tortoise. (10)
5 The body cavity of birds that makes up the thoracic and abdominal cavities. (6)
8 In birds it is the terminal end of the urinary, reproductive, and gastrointestinal tracts. (6)
10 A lizard has the ability to drop, break off, or __ part of its tail when grabbed by a predator. (10)
11 To irrigate or wash. (6)
12 The nostrils; the external openings of the nasal cavity. (5)
13 The lower or ventral shell of turtles and tortoises. (8)

Down

2 Uneven eye size. (10)
4 A small hemorrhagic spot, larger than petechiae, in the skin or mucous membrane, forming a nonelevated, rounded or irregular, blue or purplish patch. (9)
6 The upper or dorsal shell of turtles and tortoises. (8)
7 In snakes, the large scales found on the ventral aspect of the body. (6)
8 An outpocketing of the esophagus in birds. (4)
9 Referring to turtles and tortoises. (9)

29 Nursing Care of Laboratory Animals

LEARNING OBJECTIVES

After reviewing this chapter, the reader will be able to:
- Discuss how biomedical research affects the lives of people and animals
- Describe the positive and negative aspects of biomedical research
- Describe the views of the Animal Rights and the Animal Liberationists groups
- List and describe the laws that protect the public from animal abuse
- Explain the principles of the 3 Rs
- Describe the role of mice and rats in biomedical research
- State the general characteristics of mice, rats, hamsters, gerbils, guinea pigs, chinchillas, rabbits, and ferrets
- Discuss husbandry and principles of sanitation for laboratory animals
- Describe techniques for general nursing care of rodents, rabbits, and ferrets
- Describe techniques used for diagnosing and treating disease in small mammals
- List and describe methods of sample collection in laboratory animals
- State routes of administration of medication in laboratory animals
- Describe identification methods used in research animals
- Discuss anesthesia of rodents, rabbits, and ferrets

WORD PUZZLE

Answer the following questions and unscramble the letters in parentheses to reveal the hidden word.

1. Commonly used in research: (_) __ __ __ __ __

2. Type of research commonly performed: __ __ __ __ (_) __ __ __ __ __

3. A reason why Muridae species are used in research: __ __ __ __ __ (_) __ __ __ __ __

4. A common trait of muridae species: (_) __ __ __ __ __

5. A variety of strain used: __ __ __ __ (_) __

6. Acronym referring to genetically modified mice: __ (_) __

7. Example of a mutant strain: __ (_) __ __ __ __ __ __ __ __ __ __ __ __ __

8. Type of caging used to collect waste products: __ (_) __ __ __ __ __ __ __

9. Respiratory allergens common in this species: __ __ (_) __ __ __ __ __

10. DNA injected into zygote pronucleus: (_) __ __ __ __ __ __ __ __ __

Scrambled word: __ __ __ __ __ __ __ __ __ __

DEFINITIONS

Define the following:

1. Diastema _____

2. Harderian _____

3. Hystricomorph _____

4. Lagomorph _____

5. Haustra _____

6. Catabolic _____

MATCHING

Match the disease or conditions with the descriptions.

_____ 1. *Bordetella bronchiseptica*

_____ 2. Canine distemper

_____ 3. Coccidia

_____ 4. Heat stroke

_____ 5. Lymphocytic choriomeningitis

_____ 6. MHV

_____ 7. *Mycoplasma pulmonis*

_____ 8. *Pasteurella multocida*

_____ 9. Proliferative ileitis

_____ 10. Psoroptes

_____ 11. Rednose

_____ 12. Ringtail

_____ 13. *Streptococcus zooepidemicus*

_____ 14. *Syphacia* or *Aspicularis*

A. Common pinworm of mice
B. Spontaneous bacterial infection of young hamsters
C. Subcutaneous abscess or cervical lumps
D. Rabbit ear mite
E. Common endoparasite in rabbits
F. Zoonotic virus of hamsters
G. Contagious respiratory/GI disease
H. Condition of rat pups housed in low humidity
I. Nasal dermatitis associated with gerbils
J. Susceptibility in guinea pigs
K. Chinchillas are prone to this when increased humidity is present
L. "Snuffles"
M. Respiratory disease common in rats
N. Fatal disease of ferrets

FILL IN THE BLANKS

1. The maximum amount of blood that should be taken from a rat, guinea pig, or rabbit is _____ ml, while no more than _____ ml should be taken from a mouse.

2. The intravenous sites most likely used with rats include:

   a. _____

   b. _____

   c. _____

   d. _____

3. The best choices of intravenous sites for a rabbit are:

   a. _____

   b. _____

   c. _____

COMPLETE THE CHART

	Genus Species	Adult weight (grams)	Gestation (days)	Estrous cycle (days)	Body temperature °C	Life span (years)	Fill in the blank
Mice						3	Subordinate mice often show evidence of _____
Rat						2½-3½	_____ tumors are quite common
Syrian Hamster					38.9		Cheek pouches are _____
Mongolian Gerbil	*Meriones unguiculatus*			4-6	37.4-39.0	3	Female gerbil: _____
Guinea Pig						4-5	Vitamin _____ requirement
Chinchilla	*Chinchilla longer*			30-0		10	Access to a _____ should be provided as part of the husbandry
Rabbit – New Zealand White				Induced ovulator			Young are called _____
Ferret	*Mustela putorius its furo*	0.8 - 1.2 kg		Induced ovulator		5-8	Susceptible to and should be vaccinated for _____

TRUE OR FALSE

1. _____ The rat stomach has a glandular and a nonglandular portion with the esophagus following the ridge fold.

2. _____ Gerbils are permissive hibernators when the temperature is less than 8° C.

3. _____ Anogenital distance is used to differentiate male from female rats, mice, hamsters, and chinchillas.

4. _____ Hamsters can develop a vitamin C deficiency if fed old food.

5. _____ Gerbils have a large adrenal gland and increased cholesterol and lipemic serum.

6. _____ Only the male gerbil has a midventral dark orange sebaceous gland that is used for territory marking.

7. _____ Hamsters are the species most prone to spontaneous seizures.

8. _____ The sites most likely used for venipuncture for ferrets are cephalic, cranial vena cava, lateral saphenous vein, and (in large ferrets) central tail artery.

9. _____ Kurloff cells are large mononuclear lymphocytes found in conjunction with estrogen stimulation in female guinea pigs.

10. _____ Chinchillas, like guinea pigs, have open growing teeth, but unlike guinea pigs dystocia is not common.

11. _____ Ferrets have sweat glands in the skin and retractable claws.

12. _____ The sebaceous secretions found in the skin glands, not the anal glands, are responsible for the musty odor of ferrets.

13. _____ Female ferrets are prone to estrogen toxicity with bone marrow suppression and severe anemia if they are not bred once they ovulate.

14. _____ Antibiotics that are generally considered safe for guinea pigs, hamsters, and similar laboratory animals are enrofloxacin, chloramphenicol, and ciprofloxacin.

PICTURE QUIZ

1. What is this unit called, and why is it used?

_____

_____

_____

2. Is this the proper hold for an intraperitoneal injection? Why or why not?

_____

_____

_____

WORD SEARCH

Diagnostics and Treatment

Identify the term described and then find the words in the word search. When you are finished, unscramble the unused letters in the puzzle.

1. Free choice, as much as desired _____

2. A metallic element essential for the normal development and functioning of the body; an important constituent of

   bone and teeth _____

3. Antimicrobial _____

4. Of or relating to the head _____

5. Any of several mostly anaerobic Gram-positive bacteria that are present in the soil and in the intestines of humans

   and animals _____

6. Frequent passage of loose, watery stool _____

7. Antibiotic safe to use with rabbits and rodents _____

8. To supply drinking water _____

9. Decreased body temperature _____

10. Referring to route of injection directly into the marrow of the bone _____

11. Abnormal levels of certain fats accumulate in the body _____

12. Pertaining to the nose and stomach, particularly placement of a feeding tube into the stomach via the nares

    _____

13. Pasty nutritional supplement _____

14. Below the skin, as an injection _____

15. One of the many places from which a laboratory worker can withdraw blood from a mouse _____

    _____

16. Extremely overweight _____

17. When a dominant mouse chews the fur of a subordinate mouse _____

E	T	A	R	D	Y	H	T	E	N	C	M	N
V	S	U	B	C	U	T	A	N	E	O	U	S
C	U	N	U	T	R	I	C	A	L	A	I	H
E	O	A	C	A	G	I	R	R	A	L	D	Y
P	E	S	I	I	N	D	I	Y	D	I	I	P
H	S	O	T	L	I	I	C	C	L	P	R	O
A	S	G	O	V	R	A	A	A	I	I	T	T
L	O	A	I	E	E	R	L	E	B	D	S	H
I	A	S	B	I	B	R	C	E	I	O	O	E
C	R	T	I	N	R	H	I	S	T	S	L	R
E	T	R	T	H	A	E	U	E	U	I	C	M
T	N	I	N	N	B	A	M	B	M	S	I	I
N	I	C	A	X	O	L	F	O	R	N	E	A

The letters that remain form an important component involved in the care of the animals:

_ _ _ _ _ _ _ _ _ _   _ _ _ _ _ _ _ _ _

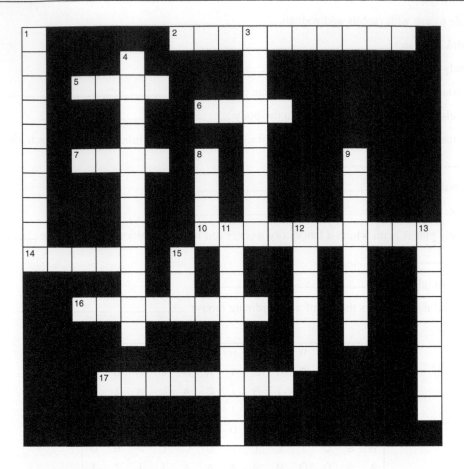

Across

2 Also known as pododermatitis, it is an inflammation of the ball of the foot of birds and guinea pigs. (10)

5 A male guinea pig. (4)

6 A male ferret. (4)

7 A male rabbit. (4)

10 Gnawing mammals that have two pairs or incisors in the upper jaw, one behind the other. (10)

14 A common name for guinea pigs. (5)

16 Loss of hair. (8)

17 Capable of being transmitted from animals to human beings. (8)

Down

1 Animals containing foreign DNA that was injected directly into the pronucleus of a zygote. (10)

3 When a dominant mouse chews the fur of a subordinate mouse. (9)

4 Improper positioning of teeth. (12)

8 A female ferret. (4)

9 Itching. (8)

11 Free choice; as much as desired. (2 words) (9)

12 Pertaining to mice or rats. (6)

13 A surveillance animal housed for the purpose of identifying abnormal occurrences. (8)

15 A female rabbit. (3)

Printed and bound by CPI Group (UK) Ltd, Croydon, CR0 4YY

03/10/2024

01040310-0016